SAFEGUARDING THE PUBLIC

Safeguarding the Public

Historical Aspects
of Medicinal Drug Control

Edited by John B. Blake

Papers from a Conference Sponsored by the
National Library of Medicine
and the
Josiah Macy, Jr. Foundation

The Johns Hopkins Press   Baltimore and London·

The Johns Hopkins Press, Baltimore, Maryland 21218
The Johns Hopkins Press Ltd., London

Library of Congress Catalog Card Number 76–84651

Standard Book Number 8018-1054-X

Contents

Part I: EUROPEAN BACKGROUNDS

Drug Control in Nineteenth-Century France:
Antecedents and Directions. *Alex Berman* 3

Drug Control in Britain, 1850–1914. *Ernst W. Stieb* 15

Drug Control in Britain: From World War I to the
Medicines Bill of 1968. *T. D. Whittet* 27

Commentary. *Melvin P. Earles* 38

Commentary. *Gert Brieger* 41

Discussion 43

Part II: SCIENTIFIC BACKGROUNDS

A Short Survey of Drug Therapy Prior to 1900.
Erwin H. Ackerknecht 51

The Appraisal of Analgesic Agents in Recent Decades:
Prototype for the Study of Subjective Responses.
Henry K. Beecher 59

The Role of the Pharmaceutical Industry. *David L. Cowen* . . 72

Commentary. *Lester S. King* 83

Commentary. *Karl H. Beyer, Jr.* 88

Discussion 91

Part III: PRIVATE PROFESSIONAL CONTROLS

Contribution of the Pharmaceutical Profession Toward
Controlling the Quality of Drugs in the Nineteenth
Century. *Glenn Sonnedecker* 97

The Prescription-Drug Policies of the American Medical
Association in the Progressive Era. *James G. Burrow* . . 112

The American Medical Association's Policy on Drugs in
Recent Decades. *Harry F. Dowling* 123

180543

Commentary. *William B. Bean* 132

Commentary. *John R. Lewis* 135

Discussion 139

Part IV: FEDERAL REGULATION

Drugs and the 1906 Law. *James Harvey Young* 147

The Evolution of the Contemporary System of Drug
    Regulation under the 1938 Act. *David F. Cavers* . . . 158

1938–1968: The FDA, the Drug Industry, the Medical
    Profession, and the Public. *Louis Lasagna*. 171

Commentary. *Vincent A. Kleinfeld* 180

Commentary. *Wallace F. Janssen*. 186

Discussion 189

Index 197

Preface

The Conference on the History of Medicinal Drug Control reported in this volume is the second on the history of medicine to be sponsored jointly by the National Library of Medicine and the Josiah Macy, Jr. Foundation. The first conference, held in 1966, addressed itself to problems of the discipline.[1] This second conference, held at the Library in Bethesda, Maryland, on May 16–17, 1968, addressed itself to one of the most pressing scientific and social problems facing medicine today.

Both conferences originated in a belief in the value of medical history shared by the Library and the Macy Foundation. This belief does not imply any expectation that this conference—or, indeed, that history itself—might come up with specific answers to practical questions of immediate policy. To claim this would be quackery no less egregious than the Cuforhedake Brane-Fude first attacked, as Dr. Harvey Young reminds us, by Dr. Wiley's Bureau of Chemistry. It is our belief that history, pursued with open-minded integrity rather than a determination to reach preconceived conclusions, can provide a perspective that enhances the understanding and judgment necessary for the wise solution of human problems. The editor hopes that readers will agree that our speakers have approached their topics in this spirit.

Each speaker was asked to consider especially problems relating to controls of the purity, quality, safety, and efficacy of drugs prescribed by physicians rather than problems relating to out-and-out quackery, narcotic control, or price control. The conference was divided into four sessions, with three speakers and two prepared discussants in each. Time was allowed at each session for free discussion, which was recorded on tape. The editor has exercised his prerogative freely to rearrange, condense, and delete parts of the transcript. In all cases the speakers have had an opportunity to review their remarks before publication. The views presented by the speakers are, of course, their own, and in no way reflect official policy of the Library or of the Department of Health, Education, and Welfare. The list of participants includes only those who are actually quoted in the published conference report.

John B. Blake

National Library of Medicine
Bethesda, Maryland

---

1. *Education in the History of Medicine.* Report of a Macy Conference sponsored by the Josiah Macy, Jr. Foundation in cooperation with the National Library of Medicine, Bethesda, Maryland, June 22–24, 1966, edited by John B. Blake (New York: Hafner, 1968).

List of Participants

Erwin H. Ackerknecht, M.D.
Professor of the History of Medicine
University of Zurich
Zurich, Switzerland

William B. Bean, M.D.
Professor of Medicine
University of Iowa
Iowa City, Iowa

Henry K. Beecher, M.D.
Dorr Professor of Research in Anaesthesia
Harvard Medical School
Massachusetts General Hospital
Boston, Massachusetts

Saul Benison, Ph.D.
Adjunct Professor
Department of History
Brandeis University
Waltham, Massachusetts

Alex Berman, Ph.D.
Professor and Chairman
Department of Historical and
    Social Studies in Pharmacy
College of Pharmacy
University of Cincinnati
Cincinnati, Ohio

Karl H. Beyer, Jr., M.D., Ph.D.
Senior Vice President
Merck Sharp & Dohme
Research Laboratories
West Point, Pennsylvania

John B. Blake, Ph.D.
Chief, History of Medicine Division
National Library of Medicine
Bethesda, Maryland

Gert Brieger, M.D., Ph.D.
Associate Professor
Institute of the History of Medicine
The Johns Hopkins University
Baltimore, Maryland

James G. Burrow, Ph.D.
Associate Professor
Department of History
Indiana State University
Terre Haute, Indiana

David F. Cavers, LL.D.
Fessenden Professor of Law
Law School of Harvard University
Cambridge, Massachusetts

Joseph D. Cooper, Ph.D.
Professor of Government
Howard University
Washington, D.C.

David L. Cowen
Professor and Chairman
Department of History
University College
Rutgers—The State University
New Brunswick, New Jersey

Harry F. Dowling, M.D.
Professor and Chairman
Department of Medicine
University of Illinois College of Medicine
Chicago, Illinois

Melvin P. Earles, Ph.D.
Professor
Department of Pharmacy
Chelsea College of Science and Technology
University of London
London, England

Don E. Francke, D.Sc.
Professor and Chairman
Department of Hospital Pharmacy
College of Pharmacy
University of Cincinnati
Cincinnati, Ohio

Benjamin Gordon
Staff Economist
U.S. Senate Small Business Committee
Washington, D.C.

Wallace F. Janssen
Historian
Food and Drug Administration
Washington, D.C.

Lester S. King, M.D.
Senior Editor
Journal of the American Medical Association
Chicago, Illinois

Vincent A. Kleinfeld
Attorney
Washington, D.C.

Louis Lasagna, M.D.
Associate Professor
Departments of Medicine (Division of Clinical Pharmacology)
  and of Pharmacology and Experimental Therapeutics
The Johns Hopkins University
School of Medicine
Baltimore, Maryland

John R. Lewis, Ph.D.
Associate Director
Department of Drugs
American Medical Association
Chicago, Illinois

Glenn Sonnedecker, Ph.D.
Professor of the History of Pharmacy
University of Wisconsin
Madison, Wisconsin

Ernst W. Stieb, Ph.D.
Professor of the History of Pharmacy
Faculty of Pharmacy
University of Toronto
Toronto, Ontario

T. D. Whittet, Ph.D.
Chief Pharmacist
Department of Health and Social Security
London, England

James Harvey Young, Ph.D.
Professor of History
Emory University
Atlanta, Georgia

Part I: European Backgrounds

Drug Control in Nineteenth-Century France: Antecedents and Directions

Alex Berman

Serious measures were taken under the *ancien régime* in France to fix responsibility for the control and distribution of drugs, to set standards for medication, to regulate the sale of secret remedies, and even to evaluate clinically the efficacy of certain medications.

By royal decree, the apothecaries of Paris were separated from the spicers in 1777 and organized into a strong corporate body, the College of Pharmacy, whose members alone were authorized to operate pharmaceutical laboratories and *officines* and to fill the prescriptions of physicians. The spicers could sell at wholesale crude, uncompounded plant drugs, using the customary weights of commerce, but not medicinal weight (*poids médicinal*). However, they were permitted to sell at retail and by medicinal weight manna, cinnamon, rhubarb, senna, and simple roots and barks. Apothecaries were empowered to file complaints and investigate the illegal practice of pharmacy. Annual inspection of drugs in apothecary shops was carried out by provosts of the College of Pharmacy and representatives of the Faculty of Medicine. The spicers were also inspected annually by the wardens of their own corporation and by members of the medical faculty. Sanctions for substandard drugs and for other infractions of the law were clearly indicated.[1]

Progress of a sort was made with the appearance of the last edition of the *Codex medicamentarius* for Paris in 1758, which had been purged by the Faculty of Medicine of some of the more bizarre drugs contained in previous editions—hair, mummy, human blood and skull, placenta, and urine—although it still retained dog, peacock, pigeon, chicken, serpent, and cow dung. Yet it was the most prestigious and most ambitious attempt to standardize and unify drugs for Paris and the suburbs and it compared favorably with other local official French pharmacopoeias or

---

This paper is derived from an extensive project now in progress entitled "Studies in Nineteenth-Century French Pharmacy," supported by a grant from the Public Health Service, National Library of Medicine (LM 00064).

1. *Codex medicamentarius Gallicus seu pharmacopoea gallica. Pharmacopée française rédigée par ordre du gouvernement.* 6th ed., 2 vols., vol. 1 (Rennes: Imp. Oberthur, 1937). The full text of the "Déclaration du Roi du 25 avril 1777" is given on pp. 6–7. This volume, which contains the main body of laws dealing with French pharmacy, will hereafter be referred to as *Codex* (1937), 1.

with the earlier nonofficial compendia of Brice Bauderon, Jean de Renou, Moïse Charas, or Nicolas Lémery, which were still in use.[2]

The monarchy also attempted to regulate the rapidly increasing growth of secret proprietary remedies. In 1728 a series of important decrees was issued, one delegating to the Lieutenant General of Police of Paris powers of surveillance over proprietary medications, another creating the first of numerous commissions to deal with this problem. The late historian of pharmacy Maurice Bouvet has pointed out, however, that by 1776 control of secret remedies was being carried on not only by the Lieutenant General of Police, but also by a Royal Commission of Medicine, the Faculty of Medicine, and even the Royal Academy of Sciences. Some medications had been purchased by the government and authorized by letters patent and special privileges of the King. There were, of course, many nostrums which were sold in contravention of the law. In 1778 the crown moved to make the newly founded Royal Society of Medicine the main authority for the approval of secret remedies. Analyses of secret remedies were made by many pharmacists, such as Louis Lémery (brother of Nicolas), Philippe Nicolas Pia, Louis Claude Cadet, Deyeux, and Bayen. Pierre Bayen, in 1768, was ordered to analyze all secret remedies used in military hospitals. Other names associated with the analyses of proprietary medications during the eighteenth century are Bucquet, Macquer, Geoffroy, Fourcroy, and Berthollet.[3]

In addition to numerous chemical analyses of secret remedies assigned to commissions and individuals, there were also attempts to determine their efficacy by means of clinical trials on the patient. Many nostrums were rejected, others accepted, by the Royal Society of Medicine before the Revolution. A case in point is one of the most flamboyant and long-lived of the eighteenth-century French nostrums, the *rob Boyveau-Laffecteur*, advertised principally as a cure for syphilis. Launched in 1764, it received its first clinical trials in military hospitals. In 1776 the physician Poissonier des Perrières tried this remedy on three soldiers at the hospital attached to the military barracks in Saint-Denis. Within two years, this concoction had received a warm reception by the medical profession. It had been tested on twelve patients from the Bicêtre, and favorable results were confirmed by doctors from the Faculty of Medicine and the Royal Society of Medicine such as Geoffroy, Darcet, Vicq d'Azyr, Paulet, and others. Chemical analyses made by Darcet and Bucquet failed to show the

2. J. Bergounioux, "Les éditions du Codex de l'ancienne Faculté de Paris," *Bull. Soc. Hist. Pharm.*, no. 57 (Jan., 1928), pp. 20–26; no. 58 (Apr., 1928), p. 76.
3. Maurice Bouvet, "Histoire sommaire du remède secret," *Rev. Hist. Pharm.*, no. 153 (June, 1957), pp. 57–63; no. 154 (Sept., 1957), pp. 109–18; "Sur l'essai des médicaments en France avant 1789," *ibid.*, no. 149 (June, 1956), pp. 305–16; "Les commissions de contrôle des spécialités pharmaceutiques au XVIIIᵉ siècle," *Bull. Soc. Hist. Pharm.*, no. 35 (July, 1922), pp. 88–94; no. 36 (Oct., 1922), pp. 119–24.

presence of mercury or other minerals. After more clinical evaluation at the Bicêtre, additional analysis by Bucquet, and further scrutiny by distinguished representatives of the Royal Society of Medicine, the *rob* was given a clean bill of health in 1780 and proclaimed a valuable remedy for venereal diseases. This final approbation marked a resounding triumph for the promoters of this nostrum; its success remained unabated for decades.[4] Clinical evaluations were also made on other proprietary medications such as the *eau médicinale* of Husson at the Invalides in 1775 and the *tisane Caraïbe* at the Bicêtre and other institutions in 1779; that same year, the physician De Horne conducted trials in three hospitals on such alleged specifics for venereal disease as the *fumigations de Lalouette, lavement de Royer, pilules de Keyser, pilules de Belloste*, and other remedies.[5]

Despite some successes, the *ancien régime* was unable to stem the alarming growth and sale of secret remedies. The *Comité de Salubrité* of the National Constituent Assembly (1790–91) attacked this problem in earnest.[6] Proposals for pharmaceutical reforms were made by the Royal Society of Medicine, by Vicq d'Azyr (1790), and by Guillotin (1791); reports were presented to the Council of Five Hundred by Braillon, Calès, and Pastoret (1797), by Barras, Vittet, and Cabanis (1798), and during the Consulate by Fourcroy and Carret (du Rhône). All this activity laid the groundwork for the reorganization of pharmacy in France and for stringent controls on drugs.[7]

The Law of Germinal, promulgated in 1803, emerged as the fundamental legislation regulating the practice of pharmacy; it was explicit and ruthless in its articles 32 and 36, which authorized only pharmacists to fill prescriptions of medical practitioners and to stock only medications listed in drug compendia approved by the schools of medicine. All remedies not meeting these requirements were considered secret and illegal. Article 36 specifically forbade the advertising, distribution, and sale of any secret remedy. Fines and imprisonment were specified in legislation passed in 1805 (Loi du 29 Pluviôse an XIII).[8]

4. Maurice Bouvet, "Un remède secret du XVIIIᵉ siècle: le rob Boyveau-Laffecteur," *Bull. Soc. Hist. Pharm.*, no. 39 (June, 1923), pp. 264–72. See also the favorable account of this remedy by Fournier-Pescay, "Rob antisyphilitique de Laffecteur," in *Dictionaire des sciences médicales*, 60 vols. (Paris: C. L. F. Panckoucke, 1812–22), 49: 60–69.

5. Maurice Bouvet, "Histoire sommaire du remède secret," p. 62.

6. Henry Ingrand, *Le Comité de Salubrité de l'Assemblée Nationale (1790–1791)*, Thesis, Paris (Paris: Librairie Médicale Marcel Vigne, 1934), pp. 73–76. See also L. Faligot, *La question des remèdes secrets sous la Révolution et l'Empire* (Paris: Occitania, 1924), pp. 28–90.

7. Faligot, *La question des remèdes secrets*, pp. 28–58; L. André-Pontier, *Histoire de la pharmacie* (Paris: Octave Doin, 1900), pp. 245–61.

8. *Codex* (1937), 1: 11–12.

It seemed that the question of secret remedies had finally been dis-
posed of in peremptory fashion. But this was not to be the case. The
first blow came on June 14, 1805 (25 Prairial an XIII), when a decree
was issued permitting the sale of all proprietary medicines that had been
officially authorized prior to the 1803 legislation with no obligation
on the part of the inventors to divulge the composition of their products.
In an effort to repair the damage, another edict was signed by Napoleon
on August 18, 1810, proclaiming that henceforth all previously approved
secret remedies, as well as any future ones, would have to be authorized
by the Minister of the Interior upon the recommendation of an appointed
commission, three of whose five members would be chosen from the
medical schools. The commission would study the composition of the
remedy, determine its safety and efficacy, and, if it was judged valuable,
recommend purchase of the formula from the inventor at a fair
price.[9]

Another decree issued four months later prolonged the term of
compliance.[10] It became apparent in the next few years that official
inertia and political vagaries would prevent the implementation of
this legislation. By 1817 the pharmacist Charles Louis Cadet de Gassicourt, then visiting London, could console himself that there were
probably more charlatans peddling nostrums in England than in France.[11]
The German physician J. L. Casper wrote in 1822 that the rampant
sale of secret remedies in Paris and London contrasted sharply with
the strict regulation in Germany.[12] An official circular issued by the
French Minister of the Interior in 1828 served only to underline the seriousness of the situation. "I have proof," stated the Minister, "that posters
are put up in the streets, that advertisements appear in the newspapers,
that pharmacies sell secret remedies for the treatment of certain diseases;
often in these advertisements authorizations are claimed which have never
been granted. . . ."[13] By 1831 at least six secret remedies had been judged
legal by the authorities: the *grains de santé du docteur Franck*, the *poudre
d'Irroë*, the indestructible *rob Boyveau-Laffecteur*, the *pommade de la veuve
Farnier*, the *pilules de Belloste*, and the dermatological preparations of
Kunckel. Also declared legal at this time, allegedly for their nonmedicinal

9. *Codex* (1937), 1:146–47. See also Maurice Bouvet, "La législation de la spécialité
pharmaceutique sous le régime de la Loi de Germinal," *Pharm. Franc.* 28 (1924): 2–9.
10. *Codex* (1937), 1:148.
11. C. L. Cadet [de Gassicourt], "De l'état de la médecine et de la pharmacie en
Angleterre," *J. Pharm. Sci. Access.* 3 (1817): 321–34.
12. J. L. Casper, *Charakteristik der französischen Medicin mit vergleichenden
Hinblicken auf die englische* (Leipzig: F. A. Brockhaus, 1822), pp. 511–12.
13. Adolphe Trebuchet, *Jurisprudence de la médecine, de la chirurgie, et de la
pharmacie en France* (Paris: J. B. Baillière, 1834), p. 366; A. N. Narodetzki, *Le remède
secret* (Paris: Librairie Générale de Droit et de Jurisprudence, 1928), pp. 26–27; Bouvet,
"La législation de la spécialité pharmaceutique," pp. 30–31.

properties, were the *pâte Regnauld* and *eau de Botot*, the former sold by the clever promoter Dr. L. D. Véron, Director of the Paris Opera and owner of the journal *Constitutionnel*, who was featured in many of Daumier's caricatures.[14] Not only Daumier lampooned secret remedies and pharmacy; a number of other prominent French caricaturists of the nineteenth century joined in—Traviès, Philipon, Charles Jacque, Grandville, Gavarni, Cham, and Vernier.[15]

In 1820 the task of approving proprietary medications shifted to the newly founded Academy of Medicine and its Commission on Secret and New Remedies. The results in subsequent years were hardly impressive. Between 1830 and 1843 the Academy recommended to the government the purchase of three secret products—*pilules de Belloste, biscuits anti-syphilitiques d'Ollivier*, and *poudre de Sency*—none of which was ever actually bought, because of lack of funds. The Academy also approved a few secret remedies without recommending purchase and refused approbation on a number of others.[16] In 1844 a law was passed forbidding the issue of patents for any medicinal preparation, but exempting processes, apparatus, and dosage forms, and any product judged nonmedicinal.[17] Six years later the Academy of Medicine was empowered to recognize the utility of any new medication by simply publishing the formula in its *Bulletin*, after receiving the approval of the Minister of Agriculture and Commerce and the consent of the inventor (*décret du 3 mai 1850*). Such a remedy then ceased to be secret and could be marketed pending its inclusion in the *Codex*.[18]

But all this legislation did not stop the profusion of proprietary medications whose legality was hotly disputed in the courts and whose existence was enhanced by a conflict of laws. From Germany in 1874 came a shrill denunciation. The historian of pharmacy Carl Frederking bemoaned the fact that France and England had created a global "*Geheim- und Patent-mittelschwindel.*" It was all the fault of free enterprise in pharmacy, he wrote, which had reduced the highly regarded pharmaceutical profession in France to charlatanry.[19] Actually, many French pharmacists were strongly opposed to secret and proprietary medicines, as is demonstrated by the resolutions passed against them in the annual pharmaceutical congresses held in French cities from 1857 to 1870, and by the pronounce-

14. Bouvet, "La législation," p. 31.

15. Paul Rabier and Louis Sergent, "La spécialité dans l'art, sa caricature au XIXᵉ siècle," *Rev. Spécialités*, 5 (Mar., 1925): 69–95; Louis Sergent and Maurice Bouvet, "Quelques documents iconographiques sur le docteur Véron, directeur de l'Opéra et spécialiste," *Rev. Hist. Pharm.*, no. 128 (Dec., 1950), pp. 136–39.

16. Bouvet, "La législation," pp. 31–33.

17. *Codex* (1937), 1: 148. Bouvet, "La législation," pp. 52–54.

18. *Codex* (1937), 1: 148. Bouvet, "La législation," pp. 54–58.

19. Carl Frederking, *Grundzüge der Geschichte der Pharmacie* (Göttingen: Vandenhoeck und Ruprecht's Verlag, 1874), pp. 80–82.

ments of distinguished leaders of the profession.[20] Certainly no aspect of
drug control in nineteenth-century France aroused more controversy and
confusion. Dechambre, writing in 1876, characterized the situation as legal
chaos.[21] For more than a century after 1803, the industrial development of
proprietary medications was in legal jeopardy because successive governments had not been able to formulate a realistic definition of what constituted a "secret remedy." A solution to this problem was reached only in
1926.[22]

A much older problem that had to be faced during the nineteenth century was the adulteration of drugs. The Parisian pharmacist L. I. Nachet
wrote in 1821 of the widespread fraudulent alteration of drugs and gave a
long list of medications that were being adulterated. He cautioned against
buying powdered drugs from wholesale druggists; he bemoaned the absence of inspectors at ports of entry and the indifference of many physicians.[23] Other prominent pharmacists were equally concerned. Bussy and
Boutron-Charlard stated in 1829 that the wars of the Revolution and the
Empire, and in particular Napoleon's Continental System, had created an
ersatz climate favorable to adulteration. In subsequent years, the port of
Marseille, traditionally a source of adulterated drugs, was transformed into
a "véritable atelier de sophistiquerie" where products such as gums, resins,
balsams, manna, opium, castoreum, and musk were grossly altered. Para-
doxically, developing science and technology, which could aid in the detection of substandard drugs, could also be used by unscrupulous persons
to palm off inferior medicinal products for private gain.[24]

In addition to the writings of Nachet and Bussy and Boutron-Charlard there were other important publications available in France during the
first half of the nineteenth century dealing in whole or in part with drug
adulteration. Worthy of mention are the treatise of A. V. Favre, *De la
sophistication des substances médicamenteuses* (1812); the *Police judiciaire
pharmaco-chimique* (1816) by E. J. B. Bouillon-Lagrange and A. Vogel,
which was a translation of W. H. G. Remer's *Lehrbuch der polizeilich-
gerichtlichen Chemie* (2d ed., 1812); N. J. B. Guibourt's renowned *Histoire
naturelle des drogues simples* (1820 and subsequent editions); the *Manuel des*

20. E. Ferrand, "Voeux de la pharmacie française exprimés par les sociétés
pharmaceutiques de France, dans leurs congrès annuels de 1857 à 1870," in *Congrès
médical de France*, 4th sess., Lyon, September, 1872 (Paris, 1873), pp. 606–8; Vidal,
"Réorganisation de la pharmacie et élévation du niveau des études professionelles,"
ibid., p. 571; Bouvet, "La législation," p. 55.

21. A. Dechambre, "Remède secret," in *Dictionnaire encyclopédique des sciences
médicales*, ed. A. Dechambre (Paris: G. Masson, P. Asselin, 1864–89), 3d Ser., 3:
371–77.

22. Narodetzki, *Le remède secret*, pp. 195–216. *Codex* (1937), 1: 149.

23. L. I. Nachet, "Sophistication," in *Dictionaire des sciences médicales* (Paris,
1812–22), 52: 152–59.

24. A. Bussy and A. F. Boutron-Charlard, *Traité des moyens de reconnaître les
falsifications des drogues simples et composées* (Paris: Thomine, 1829), pp. vii–ix.

pharmaciens et des droguistes (1821), which was a French version by J. B. Kapeler and J. B. Caventou based on an earlier German work by J. C. E. Ebermeir and adapted by the translators to the needs of the 1818 *Codex*; A. Payen and A. Chevallier's *Traité élémentaire des réactifs* (1822 and later editions); Eugène Desmarest's *Traité des falsifications* (1828); and A. L. Fée's *Cours d'histoire naturelle pharmaceutique* (1828). A major work was published by J. B. A. Chevallier at mid-century: *Dictionnaire des altérations et falsifications des substances alimentaires, médicamenteuses et commerciales* (1850), which in ensuing editions and later revisions by Ernest Baudrimont dominated the field in the last half of the nineteenth century. Five years later, Hureaux's *Histoire des falsifications des substances alimentaires et médicamenteuses* was published; in 1874, J. Léon Soubeiran's *Nouveau dictionnaire des falsifications* appeared. Probably because of the very strong chemical orientation of scientists in France, the microscope was only slowly adopted as a tool for detecting adulterated food and drugs. A. W. Blyth, the British analyst, writing later in the century, observed this tendency among continental chemists and remarked that Hureaux, for example, had scarcely mentioned the microscope.[25]

Legal measures against adulterated and substandard drugs were initiated early in the nineteenth century. Articles 29, 30, and 31 of the Law of Germinal (1803), and a decree issued in Thermidor of the same year, provided for at least one annual inspection of pharmacies, wholesale druggists, and spicers.[26] Visits were to be made by teams drawn from medical and pharmacy schools where these had been established, and in other parts of the country by medical juries made up of physicians and pharmacists. Inspectors were accompanied by police officials; substandard drugs were to be confiscated and sanctions imposed. How effectively this legislation was enforced is not entirely clear. From all indications the problem persisted, accompanied by a mounting public concern over food adulteration. In 1851 the National Assembly passed legislation containing penalties for the sale of adulterated food and drugs. No new laws dealing with this problem were forthcoming until 1905.[27]

There had been a growing interest in assaying mineral and plant drugs in eighteenth-century France. Among prominent investigators were the brothers Geoffroy, Etienne-François, and Claude Joseph; the Dean of the Paris medical faculty, Théodore Baron; and the physicians and chemists J. B. Bucquet, J. M. F. Lassone, and C. M. Cornette. These attempts at drug assaying were rather inconclusive, as were earlier ones

25. A. W. Blyth, *Foods: Their Composition and Analysis*, 3d ed. (London: Chas. Griffen & Co., 1888), p. 42.
26. François Prevet, *Histoire de l'organisation sociale en pharmacie* (Paris: Recueil Sirey, 1940), pp. 810–11.
27. Prevet, *Histoire*, p. 110. See also *J. Pharm. Chim.* 19 (1851): 383–84. *Codex* (1937), 1: 13–17.

during the seventeenth century by Jean de Renou, Claude Bourdelin, and Pierre Pomet.[28] Much progress was made during the late eighteenth and early nineteenth century by Fourcroy, Vauquelin, and their students. With the advances in chemistry, and largely through the efforts of eminent pharmacist-chemists in France and Germany, during the first half of the nineteenth century many potent substances were isolated from natural products. Sir Robert Christison, the Scottish physician and toxicologist, who went to Paris as a young man in 1820 to study analytical chemistry with the pharmacist Pierre Robiquet, enthusiastically recalled the atmosphere of excitement surrounding the early discovery of alkaloids:

> My own foremost desire was to practise Proximate Organic Analysis. This branch of chemistry had been cultivated for a few years, and only for a very few, with success, in Germany and France, and nowhere with such energy as in Paris. Only a limited number, however, of natural products had hitherto been subjected successfully to investigation. Opium, nux-vomica, and Cocculus indicus had been examined with most satisfactory results; and cinchona-bark had just been added to the list. But the great importance of these few substances; their remarkable action on vital phenomena both in health and in disease; the discovery of the constituents in which these properties reside; the marvellous intensity of action of these constituents, whether as poisons or as remedies; their beautiful crystalline appearance, especially contrasted with the unattractive appearance of the articles which yield them; their most interesting chemical relations; the complex and yet methodical processes for obtaining them; the growing expectation that the discovery of them would revolutionise and simplify pharmacy as well as even therapeutics,—all conspired to raise in me a keen desire to be at least practically acquainted with the methods of investigation.[29]

But a revolution greater than even Christison could foresee occurred later in the century with the advent of synthetic organic medicinals and biological preparations, reflecting developments in organic chemistry and the emergence of bacteriology.

Although the legal basis for a national pharmacopoeia had first been elaborated in article 38 of the Law of Germinal (1803), it was only in 1818 that the new *Codex medicamentarius sive pharmacopoea Gallica* was first published by governmental decree. It replaced the former local pharmacopoeias of Montpellier, Lyon, Lille, Bordeaux, Toulouse, Strasbourg, Nancy, and other cities, and especially the old Paris *Codex*, which still had some vogue at the beginning of the nineteenth century.[30] Compiled

28. Maurice Bouvet, "Sur l'essai des médicaments en France avant 1789," *Rev. Hist. Pharm.*, no. 149 (June, 1956): 309–11.
29. Robert Christison, *The Life of Sir Robert Christison, Bart.*, 2 vols. (Edinburgh and London: Blackwood, 1885–86), 1: 270.
30. Jean Volckringer, *Evolution et unification des formulaires et des pharmacopées* (Paris: Brandouy, 1953), p. 12.

by distinguished representatives of the Faculty of Medicine and the School of Pharmacy in Paris, the new *Codex* was intended to provide national uniform standards for drugs, obligatory for all pharmacies. Three revised editions were issued during the century, in 1837, 1866, and 1884. Long intervals between revisions, however, impaired the usefulness of the *Codex* and led to the 1850 legislation, alluded to earlier, which accorded legal recognition to "new and useful remedies" upon acceptance and publication in the *Bulletin* of the Academy of Medicine, pending official listing in a revised *Codex*. In any case, new therapeutic agents became known immediately in professional journals and in the numerous private formularies published during the nineteenth century. The most influential private formulary was doubtless that of François Magendie, which ran through many editions in the 1820's and 1830's, but other names come to mind, such as F. S. Ratier, F. Foy, A. Bouchardat, and O. Reveil.[31] Of considerable interest, too, were the official hospital formularies, which reflected the therapeutic exigencies of military and civilian hospitals.[32]

The unique legal status of the *Codex*, enhanced by the authority and distinction of its successive Commissions, gave it a special place in relation to other drug compendia. Serving on the *Codex* Commissions were such prominent persons in medicine as J. J. Leroux, P. F. Percy, N. Hallé, G. Andral, A. M. Duméril, and E. F. A. Vulpian; pharmacy was represented by, among others, L. N. Vauquelin, J. B. Caventou, P. Robiquet, J. Pelletier, E. Soubeiran, and N. J. B. G. Guibourt. Presiding over the four Commissions were, respectively, Leroux, M. J. B. Orfila, J. B. Dumas, and L. D. J. Gavarret.[33] Prefatory statements in the *Codex* invariably attempted to justify each revised edition in the light of scientific advances and newer drugs. Typical was the observation of the 1837 edition: "In no other period, perhaps, has chemistry made as much progress and undergone as many changes as in the last two decades. More powerful and precise methods of analysis revealed the composition until then unknown of a large number of substances."[34] Despite this awareness, and the inclusion of newer remedies, the *Codex* remained surprisingly tradition-bound. The 1837 *Codex*, for example, still contained such medications as a syrup made with calf lung (*Sirop de Mou de Veau*), wood louse (*Cloportes*), a *Diascordium* attributed to Fracastorius, slightly modified, containing nineteen ingredients, and, above all, perhaps the most famous

31. *Ibid.*, pp. 25–26, 31.
32. *Ibid.*, pp. 22–23.
33. *Ibid.*, pp. 160–65.
34. *Codex, pharmacopée française rédigée par ordre du gouvernement par une commission composée de MM. les professeurs de la Faculté de médecine, et de l'Ecole spéciale de pharmacie de Paris* (Paris: Béchet jeune, 1839 [reimpression of 1837 edition]), p. xi.

remedy of antiquity, *Theriaca*, reduced to only seventy-one ingredients but still retaining viper.[35]

It was generally agreed that opium was the most important ingredient in theriac. C. J. A. Schwilgué had sensibly suggested at the beginning of the century that opium in an aromatic powder base should replace theriac, but tradition was too strong to permit this.[36] The names used to describe theriac, such as *"chaos informe"* and *"monstrueux assemblage"* (Bouchardat), or *"la composition monstrueuse"* (J. B. G. Barbier, F. V. Mérat, and C. L. Cadet de Gassicourt), or *"cet assemblage bizarre"* (A. Trousseau and H. Pidoux), were applied more with awe and affection than with distaste.[37] Theriac was expunged from the French *Codex* only in 1908. The Commission, abandoning it with regret, stated: "After having held for so long a prominent place in pharmacy and therapeutics, it leaves the domain of history to be relegated to legend."[38]

The *Journal de pharmacie et de chimie* in 1893 pointed out the virtual absence of assays in the *Codex*, in contrast to certain foreign pharmacopoeias,[39] and it was only in the 1908 *Codex* that assays for identity and purity were extensively introduced for the first time.[40] More stringent measures regulating the sale of poisons had been published in an ordinance of Louis Philippe in 1846.[41] National legislation to control the manufacture and sale of serums, vaccines, and other biological products was initiated in 1895.[42] But the great wave of new legislation reflecting the rapidly changing times was to come during the first three decades of the twentieth century: more vigorous steps to repress adulteration (1905); stricter laws covering drug inspection (1908 and 1909); narcotic legislation (1916);

35. *Sirop de Mou de Veau, Cloportes*, and viper were expunged from the *Codex* in 1884; the *Diascordium* and *Theriaca* were eliminated in 1908. See "Liste générale des médicaments figurant dans les diverses éditions de la pharmacopée française," in *Codex* (1937), 1: 459–591.

36. C. J. A. Schwilgué, *Traité de matière médicale*, 2d ed., 2 vols. (Paris: Brosson, 1809), 1: 344.

37. A. Bouchardat, *Nouveau formulaire magistral*, 18th ed. (Paris: Germer Baillière, 1873), p. 90. A. Bouchardat, *Manuel de matière médicale de thérapeutique comparée et de pharmacie*, 2d ed. (Paris: Germer Baillière, 1846), p. 43. J. B. G. Barbier, *Traité élémentaire de matière médicale*, 3 vols. (Paris:.Méquignon-Marvis, 1819), 2: 487. Mérat's designation is cited by E. Bourgoin in the article "Thériaque," in *Dictionnaire encyclopédique des sciences médicales*, ed. A. Dechambre, ser. 3, 17: 174. See also C. L. Cadet de Gassicourt, "Thériaque," in *Dictionaire des sciences médicales* (Paris, 1812–22), 55: 93; A. Trousseau and H. Pidoux, *Traité de thérapeutique et de matière médicale*, 5th ed., 2 vols. (Paris: Béchet jeune, 1855), 2: 44.

38. *Codex medicamentarius Gallicus, pharmacopée française rédigée par ordre du gouvernement* (Paris: Masson, 1908), p. xviii.

39. *J. Pharm. Chim.* 27 (1893): 337.

40. Jean Volckringer, "Notice Historique," in *Pharmacopée française. Codex medicamentarius Gallicus*, 7th ed. (Paris: L'Ordre National des Pharmaciens, 1965), p. 25.

41. *Codex* (1937), 1: 52–54.

42. *Codex* (1937), 1: 176–77.

the founding of a central national laboratory in the pharmacy school in Paris for the analysis of medicinal products under the jurisdiction of the Ministry of Agriculture (1918); and a ministerial decree establishing still another national laboratory at the Faculty of Pharmacy in Paris for the use of the *Codex* Commission (1922).[43] The decree of July 13, 1926, resolved the protracted problem of secret remedies. Proprietary medicines could finally be exempt from the stigma of secrecy by full disclosure of the quantity of active ingredients and the name and place of the manufacturer on the package label.[44] Decades of needless legal obfuscation passed before this obvious solution was reached.

The rise of a pharmaceutical industry in nineteenth-century France followed in many respects the pattern of other technologically advanced countries, especially in the shift from the artisan-based operation of the *officine* to the large-scale manufacture and distribution of the factory. It had become apparent before the close of the nineteenth century that the community pharmacist did not have the facilities to produce basic chemical substances and synthetic organic compounds, or for that matter the newer prefabricated dosage forms which required a considerable investment in machine technology.[45] The 1908 *Codex* had mirrored this situation with its requirements for assays and its recognition that many of the chemical compounds officially listed could be prepared only by industry.

Scientific resources for drug evaluation became increasingly available in France as the nineteenth century progressed. Before therapeutics could be set on a scientific course, it had to draw heavily on the basic sciences, especially chemistry and physiology. Yet the famous clinician Armand Trousseau bitterly disputed this assumption in the Academy of Medicine in 1860 and later in his *Clinique médicale de l'Hôtel-Dieu* (1861 and subsequent editions): "Far from me, gentlemen, is the thought of indicting the ancillary sciences and chemistry in particular; I only condemn the exaggeration and pretensions of these sciences, their clumsy and impertinent meddling in our art."[46] The historical reasons for this empirical and skeptical attitude so characteristic of the Paris clinical school have been brilliantly analyzed by Professor Ackerknecht.[47] Among those challenging this view was the military pharmacist Antoine Baudoin Poggiale,

43. *Codex* (1937), 1: 13–20, 57. For a contemporary commentary, see *Rép. Pharm.*, 20 (1908): 409–17; 21 (1909): 318–22; 30 (1918): 29; 34 (1922): 282–83; *J. Pharm. Chim.* 26 (1922): 80.

44. *Codex* (1937), 1: 149.

45. René Fabre and Georges Dillemann, *Histoire de la pharmacie* (Paris: Presses Universitaires de France, 1963), p. 122.

46. Armand Trousseau, *Clinique médicale de l'Hôtel-Dieu de Paris*, 5th ed., 3 vols. (Paris: Baillière, 1877), 1: 3.

47. E. H. Ackerknecht, *Medicine at the Paris Hospital, 1794–1848* (Baltimore: Johns Hopkins Press, 1967).

during a debate in the Academy of Medicine: "Monsieur Trousseau repudiates the progress that physical and natural sciences have made in the last 80 years; his attacks are an absolute negation of all the work accomplished in the last 25 years, and show no gratitude to the chemists and physiologists who have devoted themselves to the study of organic chemistry and physiology. It is important consequently to combat such a dangerous opinion."[48] The same issues were debated by Alfred Stillé and Roberts Bartholow during the 1870's in the United States, with Stillé objecting that "the domain of therapeutics is, at the present day, continually trespassed upon by pathology, physiology and chemistry," and Bartholow retorting that "It is obvious that no science can be created out of empirical facts."[49] In the end, the views of Poggiale and Bartholow had to be accepted.

Drug control in nineteenth-century France was marked by striking contradictions. Although there was considerable drug legislation, the laws were inflexible, conflicting, and often not enforced. Infrequent revisions of the *Codex* prevented prompt official recognition of new and valuable therapeutic agents. The virtual absence of assays in the *Codex*, together with its conservatism, seems rather incongruous in the light of the eminence of its Commissions. There was no dearth of able pharmacists, chemists, and scientists, yet the creation of government-sponsored national laboratories for drug control had to wait until the next century. And in the twentieth century, France, like many other countries, would have to provide scientific and social solutions by then vastly more urgent and complex.

48. *Bull. Acad. Imp. Med.* 25 (1859–60): 769.
49. Cited by me in "The Heroic Approach in 19th-Century Therapeutics," *Bull. Amer. Soc. Hosp. Pharm.* 11 (1954): 327.

Drug Control in Britain, 1850–1914

Ernst W. Stieb

My personal research interests and activities relating to drug control have concentrated upon the detection and control of drug adulteration in nineteenth-century Britain.[1] While this aspect of drug control is somewhat narrower than the implicit guidelines set for this conference, the control of drug adulteration did loom large enough in the picture for me to propose that I restrict myself largely to this more limited view. For purposes of this discussion I shall take the term "adulteration" to mean any procedure that produces an alteration in strength or purity, or both, from the avowed standard of a drug, whether through intent or neglect.

Drug adulteration, of course, neither began nor ended within the time limits set for this paper (1850–1914), nor were the problems of its detection and control peculiar to Britain. Its history may be traced with ease back at least to Greco-Roman antiquity. Yet nineteenth-century Britain does provide a significant focal point for the historian of this subject, for by then science and technology had progressed sufficiently to provide more and more effective weapons for detection and social forces had become strong enough to press for legislative controls.

Britain, long a stronghold of staunch laissez-faire philosophies, yet giving way increasingly during the nineteenth century to humanitarian reforms,[2] emerged with the first comprehensive laws against adulteration, and influenced the early legislative controls in other Anglo-American countries. The period 1850–1914 does constitute an important time span for our subject. It was in 1850 that Arthur Hill Hassall (1817–94), the noted

1. This paper is based largely on Ernst W. Stieb, with the collaboration of Glenn Sonnedecker, *Drug Adulteration: Detection and Control in Nineteenth-Century Britain* (Madison: University of Wisconsin Press, 1966). The reader is referred to this publication for detailed discussions of subjects explored more superficially in this paper.

2. See for instance the divergent views expressed by such contemporary historians as Jenifer Hart, "Nineteenth-Century Social Reform: A Tory Interpretation of History," *Past and Present*, 31 (July, 1965): 39–61; J. Bartlet Brebner, "Laissez faire and State Intervention in Nineteenth-Century Britain," in Robert Livingston Schuyler and Herman Ausubel, *The Making of English History* (New York: Dryden Press, 1952), pp. 501–10; G. Kitson Clark, *The Making of Victorian England* (London: Methuen & Co., 1962), pp. 280–83. I am grateful to David L. Cowen for drawing these references to my attention. See also Stieb, *Drug Adulteration*, p. 274, n. 4.

British physician and microscopist, began his investigations of adulteration that led ultimately to legislative controls; and it was in 1914 that
perhaps the first edition of the *British Pharmacopoeia* to take full consideration of modern scientific methods for determining drug purity or quality
appeared. In some ways 1914, with the beginning of World War I,
also signaled the end of such vestiges of the nineteenth century that
remained.

The effective control of drug adulteration depends upon both the
availability of adequate scientific and technological means of detecting
adulteration and the social measures taken to ensure their application. One
without the other is largely impotent. I therefore propose to deal briefly
with both facets.

Although the application of the microscope to the detection of
adulteration stands as perhaps the most dramatic and significant example
of science and technology applied to a problem that had remained largely
unsolved during two millennia, there were by 1850 a number of other
analytical techniques and instruments available to those who wished to,
or were able to, use them. The few qualified food and drug analysts before
the last quarter of the nineteenth century were handicapped by the almost
total absence of literature on the subject in English. In 1875 appeared the
first comprehensive work in English to provide a guide for the early
analysts, the *Outlines of Proximate Organic Analysis* by Albert Benjamin
Prescott, American physician, chemist, and pharmaceutical educator of
the University of Michigan. Hassall's books had dealt primarily with the
application of a single technique, microscopy. The void was filled soon
afterward, in 1879, by the first of a series of editions stretching into the
twentieth century by the well-known British analysts Alexander Wynter
Blyth and Alfred Henry Allen. Blyth's *Manual of Practical Chemistry*
(later titled *Foods*) and particularly Allen's eventually multi-volume
Commercial Organic Analysis provide a remarkable barometer of the
techniques developing at the end of the nineteenth and the beginning of
the twentieth centuries.

For the most part these books confirm that, with a few exceptions,
even those analytical test methods that did exist were seldom applied
to detecting drug adulteration before the end of the nineteenth century.
This was a reflection not only of the development of science and technology but also of the inadequacy of many techniques, until that time,
to probe the secrets of organic materials. It is no accident, then, that
organoleptic means of detecting drug adulteration predominated during
most of the century, which still depended mainly upon drugs of vegetable
origin. There is usually a delay from the first discovery of an instrument
or technique until its application, and then a considerably longer delay
before it makes its way into the purity rubrics of the *British Pharmacopoeia*.

Organoleptic tests or macroscopic descriptions had been applied in one form or another since earliest times; they continued as the main criteria for vegetable drug standards until the *British Pharmacopoeia* of 1914. Even the physical tests involving specific gravity, solubility, and changes of state that were known prior to the nineteenth century were applied only slowly to controlling drug adulteration. Although physical constants based upon these tests appeared earlier, it is not until 1914 that we find in the *British Pharmacopoeia* a definition of specific gravity and directions for determining melting and boiling points. Standard viscosimeters appeared in the nineteenth century, but the measure of viscosity as a determinant of quality was first seen only in the 1932 *BP* (although in the *USP* of 1916).

Among the optical techniques, colorimetry found little use during the nineteenth century, although Duboscq had developed the colorimeter in 1854. The first practical spectroscope appeared in 1859 and was first applied about a decade later. Wollaston had at once realized the applications to detecting adulteration when he made the first modern refractometer in 1802; but it was only slowly, after the more accurate Abbe refractometer appeared in 1874, that refractive indices began to receive the attention they deserved. The trend is clear in the third (1899) edition of Allen's work. Refractive indices first appeared in the 1914 *Pharmacopoeia*, which also recognized optical rotation as a valuable analytical aid. As in the case of Wollaston and the refractometer, Biot had used his first polarimeter of 1840 to detect adulteration, yet not until the blossoming of research in resins and essential oils at the turn of the century was the over-all importance of optical rotation as an analytical tool realized fully.

Among the optical instruments, the microscope provided one of the most reliable and quickly accepted means of determining food and drug purity. Instruments corrected for spherical and chromatic aberrations already existed in the first quarter of the nineteenth century. Isolated references to its use appeared before 1850, but it was really from then on, in the hands of Arthur Hill Hassall, that the microscope found comprehensive and systematic application as the first reliable means of detecting adulteration in many vegetable drugs. For this reason microscopy assumed a most important role in the history of nineteenth-century drug control; indeed, its importance increased as microscopy was coordinated with polarimetry and spectroscopy.

In the realm of chemical methods of analyses, we already find systematization in the 1840's and 1850's, as far as inorganic tests are concerned, through the work of men such as Fresenius, Gay-Lussac, and Mohr. To the extent that they could be applied to drugs of the time, inorganic test methods increased noticeably in editions of the *British Pharmacopoeia* between 1864 and 1914. But organic analysis, particularly as it relates to food and drug standards, is a child of the last quarter of the nineteenth century, as the books of Prescott, Allen, and Blyth amply testify. Even younger is biological standardization, whose merits were still being actively discussed in the late nineteenth and early twentieth centuries. Biological standards first found their way into the *British Pharmacopoeia* of 1932 (and the *USP* of 1916).

For the most part, however, the number of persons who *were* able to use any of these techniques we have referred to, and particularly in their special application to the detection of adulteration, remained small until after 1874 when the Society of Public Analysts was founded to devote special attention to the needs created by the first Adulteration Acts. A role in developing the science of food and drug analysis was also played by members of the Pharmaceutical Society of Great Britain (founded 1841) and particularly those pharmacists who also supported the British Pharmaceutical Conference (founded 1863). Yet the Conference long remained an organization of modest membership and activities, while the Pharmaceutical Society was hampered in its efforts to solve the problems of adulteration by raising the educational standards of pharmacy. The Society's best intentions were for a time thwarted by its failure to gain responsibility for a compulsory curriculum until 1908 and by postpone-ment of its full control over pharmaceutical practice until 1933. Moreover, while its school early put emphasis upon a scientific curriculum that equipped its graduates to be competent or to make worthwhile contribu-tions, only a relatively small number of practicing pharmacists took advantage of that opportunity.

The few persons equipped to deal effectively with drug adulteration during the nineteenth century were further fettered by the status and stature of the most logical set of drug standards available, the *British Pharmacopoeia*. Not only was the *Pharmacopoeia* not a statutory authority under Food and Drug Acts in Great Britain—though it became of neces-sity a presumptive standard for the courts and public analysts[3]—but its scientific competency to serve as an adequate standard was questioned increasingly during the nineteenth and into the twentieth century.

Yet the detection and control of adulteration became more and more a reality as science and technology were applied to the problem by a few motivated and concerned persons. It remained, then, for certain individuals to become sufficiently concerned and motivated to press for societal controls.

When Fredrick Accum (1769–1838) raised a muckraker's cry for control early in the century with his *Treatise on Adulterations* (1820), he

---

3. "The British Pharmacopoeia," in *The Calendar of the Pharmaceutical Society of Great Britain, 1951–1952* (London), p. 78; and Douglas C. Bartley, *Adulteration of Food: Statutes and Cases* (London: Stevens & Sons, 1895), p. 59.

created a sensational ripple, but the British spirit of laissez faire was still strong enough to offset the growing spirit of reform and humanitarianism. Accum's followers, armed with scientific weapons and buttressed by a growing concern for public health, encountered greater success, though slowly, during the second half of the century. That is not to say that various degrees of opposition, including accusations of exaggeration, were not levied against Hassall and his contemporaries in food and drug reform—the Birmingham surgeon and apothecary John Postgate (1820–81), and Thomas Wakley (1795–1862), crusading editor of the *Lancet* and reforming member of Parliament. But the social and political climate was changing, and their perseverance did find reward, though not as quickly or in as decisive a manner as they might have preferred.

That drug adulteration existed was not disputed. What was disputed was its extent and nature, its definition, who was responsible for it, and the manner in which it should be controlled. The reformers themselves did not always agree on such questions, nor did those within government or the professions.

In evaluating the extent of drug adulteration in nineteenth-century Britain, we are faced with so many qualifications that, in terms of our own period of proliferating statistics, we feel uneasy about how few of the nineteenth-century data we can honestly consider unbiased, factual, or significant. Prior to 1876, when the first regular annual reports of the Local Government Board began to appear, most statements concerning the extent of drug adulteration tended to be general and qualitative rather than specific and quantitative. Exceptions were the publications by Hassall in the 1850's and by the pharmacist Richard Phillips in the 1840's, yet both involved a relatively small number of drugs. Whatever the shortcomings of these sources and the disagreement among expert witnesses before various Parliamentary select committees (1855, 1856, 1874, 1878–79, 1894, 1895, 1896), it would appear that while drug adulteration, like food adulteration, was fairly extensive during the first half of the nineteenth century, the problem began to abate by mid-century and improved considerably as the century progressed. Objectivity is colored by the small number of drug samples actually examined by analysts before the end of the century and by the fact that such samples often tended to be those against which a case could be established with fair certainty, including some whose technical state of adulteration was open to serious question at the time. In any case, adulteration practices seem to have become less extensive as the century wore on and as they could be detected with greater certainty by the advances in science and technology to which we have already alluded.

Since the interpretation of extent of adulteration depended upon the definition of adulteration and the availability of adequate drug standards, we may more readily understand disagreements over extent when we realize fully the inadequacies during the nineteenth century of both definitions and standards. Those inadequacies hampered effective government control of adulteration and affected the legal sanctions the government was willing to impose.

Such questions as extent, nature, definition, and form of control also proved perplexing to the professions most concerned with drug adulteration, that is, medicine and pharmacy. The general attitude of the professions was the predictable one that they would prefer control to be voluntary and under their own jurisdiction rather than enforced by government action. Although the stand of the professions, particularly pharmacy, sometimes seemed compromising, it must be understood within their philosophy that drug adulteration was in many ways an internal problem which they felt capable of solving as such. That the government at first agreed is evident from the exclusion of drugs from the first British Adulteration Act of 1860.

From the time of its founding in 1841, the Pharmaceutical Society did pay considerable attention to drug adulteration and its control. It saw a solution mainly in terms of better qualified practitioners—that is, through better pharmaceutical education—and in the control of unqualified dealers in drugs. However, as we noted, the Society did not gain control over a compulsory curriculum until 1908, and its control over drugs sold by dealers other than pharmacists registered under the Society extended only to poisons under the Pharmacy Act of 1868.[4] Under section 24 of the Act of 1868 the Society of its own volition extended the 1860 Adulteration Act to medicines, while section 4 of the 1872 amendment to the 1860 Act incorporated the whole of the 1868 Pharmacy Act. Nevertheless, the Society's sphere of power was relatively narrow, and the early Adulteration Acts were virtually unenforced. During the brief interval from 1872 to 1875 the *British Pharmacopoeia* achieved status as a legal standard under the 1872 amendment by virtue of the incorporation of the Pharmacy Act, section 15 of which required adherence to the *Pharmacopoeia* for preparations contained therein. The Sale of Food and Drugs Act of 1875 repealed earlier legislation and placed drugs with foods under the same controls, although it avoided the term

4. "The Pharmaceutical Society of Great Britain: Historical Introduction," *The Calendar of the Pharmaceutical Society of Great Britain, 1917* (London), p. 25. An interesting study of medical and pharmaceutical reform movements in terms of nineteenth-century British political philosophy has been made by David L. Cowen, "Liberty, Laissez-faire and Licensure in Nineteenth Century Britain," presented as part of the symposium, "Some Interrelationships of Pharmacy and Medicine," sponsored by the American Institute of the History of Pharmacy at the meeting of the American Association for the History of Medicine, St. Louis, Mo., April 18, 1968, and at the meeting of the American Pharmaceutical Association, Miami Beach, Fla., May 6, 1968.

"adulteration" and set no standards. Although the *Pharmacopoeia* ceased to be official under food and drug legislation at that time, it continued until 1933 to be the requisite guide under the Pharmacy Act.

It is clear from its publications that members of the British Medical Association were conscious of the problems of drug adulteration; yet they seem for the most part to have been occupied with other matters. They recognized control of the problem to be within the domain of the Pharmaceutical Society and were frankly critical of the methods used by the *Lancet's* Analytical Sanitary Commission to expose adulteration practices.

While organized pharmacy thus seemed powerless to keep the problem within its jurisdiction, and while organized medicine seems to have remained largely uninvolved, individual members of the professions, primarily physicians, carried forward the crusade with zeal and resolve. We should speak briefly in this connection of Hassall, Postgate, and Wakley.

In his own way, each man made a particular contribution to the cause; together, their activities eventually resulted in success that might not have come from one pursuing the goal alone. Of the three, Arthur Hill Hassall perhaps stands out, just as Harvey W. Wiley did in the early movement for pure foods and drugs in the United States.

That Hassall's views on adulteration and its control were considered seriously is clear from his voluminous testimony before the Parliamentary select committees on adulteration, especially the first ones of 1855 and 1856, when he appeared as first and last witness and was singled out for attention in the committee report. His influence upon writers on the subject in Britain and abroad can be readily documented. Although his prominence at home may have been put to the test somewhat by public controversy, involving Wakley and others, over Hassall's contributions, capabilities, and opinions, the ultimate evaluation of his importance, in my opinion, remains unaffected:

> Hassall was first to realize full and systematic application of microscopy to the detection of adulteration. This application opened to analytical science a whole area of organic substances, and particularly drugs, that had necessarily remained previously unexplored in the light of existing chemical knowledge. Hassall, therefore, first provided a certain means of detecting adulteration, detection having previously been limited largely to inorganic chemical compounds. This meant that legal controls of adulteration could be applied effectively for the first time.[5]

Whatever Hassall's contributions, his first publication on the adulteration of coffee might possibly have remained an isolated contribution had not Thomas Wakley offered the pages of his controversial journal, the *Lancet*, as an outlet for Hassall's talents. It is in the pages

5. Stieb, *Drug Adulteration*, pp. 175–76.

of the *Lancet*, under the heading "Analytical Sanitary Commission," that Hassall first published between 1851 and 1854 his remarkable series of detailed reports on the microscopic examination of foods and drugs. While there were some criticisms of the reports and of the *Lancet*, the reports did attract wide attention.

Hassall's growing zeal for the cause was buttressed and matched by Wakley's own courage and dedication to reform, especially medical reform, of which he was a strong proponent in and out of Parliament. Yet for all the zeal and supporting evidence Hassall and Wakley could muster, their activities alone might not have led to the Parliamentary select committees of 1855 and 1856 or to the legislation that followed had not equal zeal and dedication been shown by John Postgate. Postgate's agitation for the control of food and drug adulteration sprang from the distressing practices he noted in Birmingham, with its contributing factors of urbanism and industrialism. Through meetings he organized in Birmingham and surrounding towns he made the public aware of the problem and earned the support of the Birmingham members of Parliament, William Scholefield and George Frederick Muntz. Scholefield gained the appointment and served as chairman of the Select Committee of the House of Commons that led ultimately, after numerous bills, to the first Adulteration of Food and Drink Act in 1860.

While Postgate openly regarded himself as the sire of the 1860 Act, he surely could not have succeeded without the significant testimony and scientific evidence of Hassall or the open forum for the cause that Wakley's *Lancet* supplied. Hassall provided the ammunition, Wakley the artillery, and Postgate, with the assistance of Scholefield, the means of hitting the target—legislation to control food and drug adulteration. However, their success can perhaps be described at best as limited during the course of the nineteenth and early twentieth centuries.

The first Adulteration Acts of 1860 and 1872 were entirely voluntary, since they left it up to local authorities whether or not to appoint inspectors or analysts. In spite of this rather hit-and-miss administration, the Acts do seem to have been somewhat deterrent. Greater uniformity and compliance were recognized to be desirable, however, and consequently the 1875 Act required the appointment of analysts and inspectors.

The Local Government Board was empowered to appoint analysts where local authorities had failed to do so after a reasonable period of time. Even so, the execution of the Act seems to have varied considerably from one area to another, and it was 1899 before the Board gained the power to direct analysts and inspectors to investigate the uniformity of compliance. It was also 1899 before the Board received authority to spell out the prerequisites of competency for analysts under the Act. Part of the difficulty of ensuring greater uniformity of compliance rested in the reluctance, stemming from long-standing disagreements, to give over-riding authority for administering the Acts to one central authority. With certain variations, Hassall, Postgate, and Wakley had all favored such a central authority. Yet while the Local Government Board became that authority, it lacked meaningful power during the nineteenth century. The need for some independent authoritative court of reference to resolve conflicting analytical reports had also been emphasized repeatedly, especially by the Society of Public analysts. Again, it was only after 1899 that the Society found it possible to accept the scientific adequacy of the designated court, the laboratory of the Department of Inland Revenue at Somerset House, which did not receive independent departmental status until 1911.

While some problems were perhaps to have been expected during the early stages of administration of the Adulteration Acts, many of the difficulties encountered during the nineteenth century might have been avoided. These tended to center about inadequate definitions and standards of purity, both vital to determining the nature and extent of adulteration as far as analysts and the courts were concerned. Suggestions relative to definitions and standards had been made by the Society of Public Analysts and others while the Act of 1875 was still being framed, but these suggestions were generally not followed.

In an effort to avoid possible confusion of adulteration with substitution, impurities, and accidental contamination, most legal definitions incorporated intent as an essential component of adulteration. Unfortunately the proof of such intent proved a greater stumbling block to administering the Acts than had been anticipated. The Acts of 1860 and 1872 both required the prosecutor to prove guilty knowledge or willful intent to adulterate on the part of the accused, requirements that made the Acts virtually unenforceable. The Act of 1875, perhaps taking a cue from the Pharmacy Act of 1868, retained the connotations of knowledge and intent, but shifted to the defendant responsibility to prove lack of such knowledge "with reasonable diligence."

Furthermore, lack of guilty knowledge was not considered admissible as a defense in those sections of the 1875 Act that forbade the sale of a drug to the "prejudice" of the purchaser on the grounds that it was "not of the nature, substance, and quality of the article demanded," or that it was not compounded "in accordance with the demand of the purchaser." The onus of proving innocence by virtue of exceptions again fell squarely upon the defendant.

"To the prejudice of the purchaser" now proved a phrase almost as bothersome to the administration of the law as had the earlier passages relating to proof of guilty knowledge. It required an 1879 amendment to the earlier Act to establish that it was not necessary to prove a drug defective in all three respects listed and that it was not admissible to claim that samples sold to inspectors for analytical purposes were not to the prejudice of the purchaser.

Just as the British legislature had seemed reluctant to set forth clear definitions of adulteration—indeed, the 1856 select committee had considered it "impossible to frame an enactment on this subject which [would] rely on strict definitions"[6]—so they also skirted the necessity for legal standards of purity or quality. With the 1899 amendment to the 1875 Act, provision was made for defining certain limits with respect to some dairy products, but drug standards under laws controlling adulteration had legal recognition only briefly, and almost by accident. We have already noted how the incorporation of the 1868 Pharmacy Act in the Adulteration Act of 1872 brought this about, only to be negated by the Act of 1875.

Eminent persons argued that adopting the *British Pharmacopoeia* as a statutory standard under the Act would place undue restrictions upon the sale of drugs, whereas others, equally eminent, spoke out for the need for such a standard, if necessary by incorporating section 15 of the Pharmacy Act (1868), as had been done in 1872. Acceptance of the *Pharmacopoeia* as a legal standard would also have cleared the way for a more meaningful definition of drug adulteration, a definition like that which had been advocated by the Society of Public Analysts during the last quarter of the nineteenth century. Unheeded in Britain, the Society's proposed definition, in one form or another, had become part of many of the early adulteration laws in the United States and Canada. According to the definition, a drug was considered to be adulterated:

1. If when retailed for medicinal purposes under a name recognised in the British Pharmacopoeia it [was] not equal in strength and purity to the standard laid down in that work.
2. If when sold under a name not recognised in the British Pharmacopoeia it differ[ed] materially from the standard laid down in approved works on Materia Medica, or the professed standard under which it [was] sold.[7]

With or without statutory drug standards, analysts and courts trying to work within the ground rules set by the Act were forced to establish for themselves some frames of reference. They did so by interpreting the Act to mean that, where no legal standards existed, it was incumbent upon the courts to set for themselves standards relevant to the situation.[8] Consequently, the *British Pharmacopoeia* became the presumptive

6. Great Britain, Parliament, House of Commons, Select Committee on Adulteration of Food, Drinks, and Drugs, *Report* (1856), p. vii.
7. "Proceedings of the Society of Public Analysts," *Chem. News* 31 (1875): 59.
8. Bartley, *Adulteration of Food*, p. 59.

standard for the drugs and drug preparations contained therein. As one
authority put it, "The standard of the British Pharmacopoeia is not
conclusive, but . . . very strong evidence is necessary to displace it."[9]

How good a standard the *Pharmacopoeia* provided was another matter.
When the first *British Pharmacopoeia* appeared in 1864, it was intended
to obviate some of the difficulty of operating under three different compendia, those of London, Edinburgh, and Dublin. Criticisms levied against
the earlier works were now directed toward the new one and increased
steadily as the century advanced. The main dissatisfaction lay in the
failure of the *Pharmacopoeia* to keep up with the latest advances of science
in devising the most accurate drug standards possible. The barrage of
published critiques, many lengthy, dealing with the *Pharmacopoeia* of
1898 is particularly noteworthy, and may be considered responsible in
part for the discernible change in the edition of 1914. Some of this change
may also be attributed to the increasing role played in revisions of the
Pharmacopoeia by certain members of the Pharmaceutical Society and the
Society of Public Analysts.

Because their day-to-day activities were governed by conditions set
down by food and drug legislation, probably no group was more aware
of the strengths and weaknesses of that legislation as far as controlling
the adulteration of drugs was concerned than the Society of Public
Analysts. Although the Society came into being partly to defend public
analysts working under the Acts from what they considered unwarranted
criticisms, it always had a more positive aim than simple mutual protection.
Its primary objectives and achievements were improving the competency
of public analysts and the methods for detecting adulteration, and thereby
making the laws relating to adulteration as efficient as possible. The
fact that the Society's efforts to share the collective thoughts and strengths
of its members with the government often went unrewarded during the
nineteenth century does not detract from the major credit it must receive
for whatever success the legislative controls may have had. The contributions of the Society's members to the burgeoning science of food and drug
analysis is clear from publications in the Society's own journal, the
Analyst, and elsewhere.

The Society of Public Analysts played an important role in the
control of drug adulteration in Britain during part of the period we have
been considering here, 1850 to 1914. The effectiveness of that role depended upon the advances that had taken place during the century in
science and technology and the application of these to drug control. That
control also depended upon the growing acceptance by government of

9. William James Bell, *The Sale of Food and Drugs Acts*, 7th ed., eds. Charles F.
Lloyd and R. A. Robinson (London: Butterworth, 1923), p. 30.

its social responsibilities, as pointed out by concerned men such as Hassall, Wakley, and Postgate. British laissez faire and humanitarianism both affected the process. In 1914 many perplexing problems relating to drug control remained, but progress had been made, and the experiences, even the frustrations, of the preceding decades had been instructive at home and abroad.

Drug Control in Britain: From World War I to the Medicines Bill of 1968

T. D. Whittet

The period under consideration is a particularly important one in the development of controls over the standards of drugs in Great Britain. It begins with the publication of the 1914 edition of the *British Pharmacopoeia* (the *"BP"*), a volume which represented a transitional stage between traditional remedies and modern effective drugs, and ends with the discussion in Parliament of a bill which will greatly strengthen the control of drugs and profoundly affect the practice of pharmacy.

There are three means whereby the quality of drugs is controlled in Great Britain: the standards of the *British Pharmacopoeia*, the drug testing scheme of the National Health Service, and several different laws.

The Effect of the *British Pharmacopoeia* on Drug Quality

To understand the effect of the *British Pharmacopoeia*, it is necessary to explain its legal status. The Medical Act of 1858 set up the General Medical Council and charged it with the task of publishing a British pharmacopoeia which was to replace those of London (first edition, 1618), Edinburgh (first edition, 1699), and Dublin (first edition, 1793), which had hitherto been in use in England and Wales, Scotland, and Ireland, respectively. A committee (later called commission) was formed to undertake the task, and editions were published in 1864, 1867, 1885, and 1898, with a few addenda between editions. The *British Pharmacopoeia* has had, up to the present, no legal backing, but under the British system of "case law," it is the presumptive legal standard for any drugs or preparations it contains.

The 1914 edition, although containing many traditional remedies taken from the London and other pharmacopoeias which had been handed down from much earlier times, showed many advances over the 1898 edition. The latter volume had contained a few organic chemicals, but that of 1914 introduced many more, including such important drugs as adrenaline (epinephrine), aspirin, the first barbiturate, barbitone (barbital), the first synthetic local anesthetic, and the first synthetic urinary antiseptic, hexamine (methenamine). The new edition also increased the numbers of crude drugs and pure chemicals for which assays were required.

Degrees of comminution of powders were controlled by sieve numbers. A few injections appeared, but no methods of sterilization were suggested and there were no requirements for sterility. No vaccines or sera were included because it had not yet been possible to devise standards for them. The Pharmacopoeia Committee had recommended in 1909 to the General Medical Council that it "approach the Government with a suggestion for the establishment of a public institution for the pharmacological standardisation of potent drugs and of serums." It appears that it was not possible to do this in time for the 1914 *Pharmacopoeia*.

Although World War I hindered the development of the *Pharmacopoeia* and of legislation, it caused the first biological testing of a drug to be undertaken in Great Britain. The antisyphilitic drug arsphenamine, then known as Salvarsan, had been discovered by Ehrlich in Germany in 1907 and had been imported from there until the outbreak of war. The Board of Trade issued licenses to manufacture arsphenamine to certain approved British firms, and among the conditions for granting such a license was that samples of each batch, before being put on the market, must be submitted to the Medical Research Council for testing and must pass their tests. Strangely enough, testing of German arsphenamine, when it became available again after the war, was not required. However, the part played by the Medical Research Council in the testing of arsphenamine was one of the factors leading to the passing of the first Therapeutic Substances Act in 1925, as we shall see later.

By the time the next edition of the *BP* appeared in 1932, the Therapeutic Substances Act was in force, and biological assays were included for several newly introduced drugs such as antitoxins, sera, tuberculin, organic arsenicals, posterior pituitary, and insulin. They were also required for some older drugs such as digitalis and strophanthus and their preparations and strophanthin. This edition also considerably extended the requirements for identity and purity tests and assays. An appendix appeared on sterilization methods, and tests for sterility were imposed. There were also tests for the alkalinity of the glass of ampoules.

A new edition of the *British Pharmacopoeia* was to be published every ten years from 1932, but World War II intervened and the next edition did not appear until 1948. Seven addenda, however, appeared between the two editions. Some of these dealt with wartime emergencies, but in others new drugs were introduced and important changes were made. For example, the first *Addendum* included biological assays for a number of vitamin preparations; the fourth made drastic changes in the sterilization processes; while the seventh introduced the first spectrometric method of assay and included a general monograph on tablets, with a disintegration test.

The 1948 edition introduced assays for both tablets and injections, micromethods of analysis, microscopical methods for identifying powdered crude drugs, and the pyrogen test for large-volume injections. At the time of publication it was announced that future editions would be produced every five years. An *Addendum* of 1951 made blood products official for the first time, while the 1953 edition improved the standardization of some analytical procedures, thus giving them greater precision. The *Addendum* of 1955 included an improved pyrogen test based on a sequential method; the 1958 edition introduced nonaqueous and electrometric titration methods.

In the 1963 edition the ultraviolet and infrared methods were adopted for the examination of steroids and other complex organic compounds. Chromatographic methods also made their first appearance. An *Addendum* in 1964 contained many improvements for assay methods and also revised the sterility tests. Another, of 1966, added seventy-two new monographs and adopted a new style of expression for the potency requirements of antibiotics and their preparations, designed to improve the precision of assay and to reduce the possibility of variation of activity of preparations.

The *British Pharmaceutical Codex*

In 1907 the Pharmaceutical Society of Great Britain published the first edition of the *British Pharmaceutical Codex*, which has a much wider scope than the *Pharmacopoeia*. Under case law the *Codex* has become the presumptive standard for preparations described in it but not included in the *Pharmacopoeia*. Other editions were published in 1911, 1923, 1934, 1949, 1954, 1959, and 1963.

The 1934 edition introduced qualitative standards for dressings, and that of 1949, standards for blood products. Surgical ligatures and related products were introduced in the Sixth Supplement to the 1934 volume, published in 1944. The 1963 edition gave concise definitions of terms for storage conditions and for numerous other terms such as "freshly prepared" and "recently prepared." These should help to conserve the activity of many products.

Like the *Pharmacopoeia*, the *Codex* is kept continuously under review, and there is close collaboration between the committees producing the two volumes, many members serving on committees of both organizations. In 1963 the new editions of the two books were published simultaneously, and this policy is to continue. The *Pharmacopoeia* and the *Codex* are widely used in Commonwealth countries, where they are usually officially recognized.

In 1953 the Pharmaceutical Society published the *British Veterinary Codex*, and this has become the presumptive standard for veterinary drugs and preparations in Great Britain and the Commonwealth. A supplement appeared in 1959 and a new edition in 1965.

The National Health Service Drug-Testing Scheme

In 1911 the National Health Insurance Act made insurance against sickness compulsory for wage-earners with an income below a specified figure, which was subsequently raised on several occasions until the whole community was included in the National Health Service Act of 1946. Insured persons (but not their dependents, before 1946) were entitled to free medicines and certain appliances, including dressings. Thus the state became, indirectly, the purchaser of many drugs and preparations from pharmacists. Presumably at the instigation of the Treasury or its auditors, a drug-testing scheme was introduced. It was organized by the then new Ministry of Health and consisted of the local Medical Officer of Health taking samples by purchase or on prescription forms. The samples were sent for analysis to the so-called public analysts, who in fact are usually private analysts under contract with public authorities.

This scheme was greatly disliked by pharmacists, for two principal reasons. The first was the lack of uniformity in sampling and testing, and the second that in doubtful cases prosecutions were made in open court. Even if the case failed, as many did, the proceedings were often reported in local newspapers, giving unwelcome and frequently undeserved adverse publicity.

In 1925 the Retail Pharmacists' Union (now the National Pharmaceutical Union) approached the Ministry of Health, requesting a scheme that would be more equitable to all concerned. A new scheme drawn up by the Ministry in consultation with the Union was introduced in 1925. It consisted of a test prescription written by a health insurance doctor and presented by an agent of the local Insurance Committee to the pharmacist for dispensing. The agent divided the sample into two parts, one of which was sent to the public analyst for analysis. The other was left with the pharmacist for him to have analyzed if the official sample proved to be wrong. The results were reported to the Pharmaceutical Services Sub-Committee of the local Insurance Committee, which took the action considered appropriate in each individual case. Later it was found necessary for the sample to be divided into three parts, the third being for analysis by a referee in the case of a dispute between the analysts who examined the other samples. The referee was usually the Government Chemist's laboratory. This scheme continued until World War II, when it was discontinued for the duration.

Shortly after the introduction in 1948 of the National Health Service, it was decided to reintroduce a drug-testing scheme, and a model scheme to test the dispensing of pharmacists under their terms of service was started in 1949. It included a list of drugs and a limited list of appliances which it was thought a public analyst was capable of testing. The agent of the Executive Council (the successor of the local Insurance Committee) took this list to a doctor and asked him to provide a prescription for a preparation containing drugs in this list. The doctor was obliged by his terms of service to do this, although the medical profession disliked doing so. Preparations not in the model scheme could be tested if the Executive Council had previously consulted the public analyst about his capability to do so, but this was rarely done. The procedure after dispensing was similar to that of the old scheme. Later the list of drugs was replaced by one of preparations. The aim was to test every contractor every two years.

The scheme became increasingly unsatisfactory as proprietary preparations became increasingly used. Eventually only very few of the preparations dispensed were being tested, and it became easy for a pharmacist to detect a test prescription. From the late 1950's the scheme was modified to bring in the majority of proprietary preparations, until about 85 per cent of all dispensing was being tested. In 1966, when new terms of service were being negotiated for medical practitioners, their representatives asked to be relieved of the task of providing test prescriptions; a new scheme thus had to be devised which started in May of that year. In the new scheme the inspectors of the Pharmaceutical Society take samples of dispensed preparations awaiting collection by patients and send them for analysis in the usual way.

In the old scheme about 7,000 samples were tested annually, and the incidence of errors was 0.8 per cent in 1951 to 0.6 per cent in 1955. Figures have not been available since then. Since some of these errors were trivial, the system represents a good standard of accuracy of dispensing by the pharmacist contractors.

Legal Control of Drug Quality

At the beginning of the period under discussion, the only law concerned with the purity or quality of drugs was the Food and Drugs Act of 1875, which had a very limited scope. In 1920 the Minister of Health set up a committee "to consider and advise upon the legislative and administrative measures to be taken for the effective control of the quality and authenticity of such therapeutic substances offered for sale to the public as cannot be tested adequately by direct chemical means."

The committee interpreted the term "therapeutic substance" to include prophylactic and diagnostic agents as well as purely curative substances. They considered that the substances within their terms of reference fell into three groups:

(A) A group comprising the bodies conveniently described in the United States Regulations of 1919 as "biologic products," *i.e.*, vaccines, sera, toxins, antitoxins and analogous products.

(B) A group of potent synthetic remedies such as Salvarsan and its analogues.

(C) A group corresponding more nearly with the popularly received definition of ordinary "drugs," *e.g.*, preparations of Digitalis, Strophanthus, Squill, Ergot, Cannabis Indica, Pituitary Gland, &c. . . .

The substances in Group A cannot be tested either for purity, potency, or authenticity by chemical means. These products are liable in the process of manufacture to bacterial contamination, which must be detected by other than chemical means, and they cannot safely be sterilized by heat or by chemical agencies without seriously impairing their efficiency. They are given, not by mouth, but by means of hypodermic, intramuscular, intrathecal, or intravenous injection. Their purity, potency, and authenticity are therefore matters of vital importance . . . .

Substances in Group B are synthetic chemicals, of which the chemical, composition of the main product is known: but experience has demonstrated that slight and unappreciated variations in the process of manufacture may produce such variations in their properties as to render them highly toxic. The margin between therapeutic efficiency and dangerous toxicity is in any case a narrow one and can only be ascertained by other than chemical means. An efficient test is the more essential since the usual method of administration of these substances is by intravenous injection.

Group C is sharply differentiated from both the preceding groups and in it are included the only substances, coming within our terms of reference, which are habitually given by the mouth. Most of the substances in this group are already included in the British Pharmacopoeia, and certain primitive tests and methods of identification are therein provided for them. There is, however, an important body of professional opinion that these tests are far from adequate as standards of therapeutic efficiency. . . .

The Committee took evidence concerning the methods adopted to control the purity and authenticity of products of the same nature in the United States and Germany. Their report was issued in 1921. The following is a summary of their recommendations:

(a) That therapeutic substances which cannot be tested adequately by chemical means should be subject to supervision and control.

(b) That the Controlling Authority should be the Committee of the Privy Council. . . . [Its] main functions . . . should be to decide from time to time what substances are to be brought under control, and to prescribe the methods of standardisation and testing for these substances.

(c) That the Controlling Authority should be assisted by an Advisory Committee. . . .

(d) That there should be a Central Laboratory under Government control, wherein standards would be prepared and maintained, research carried out in connection therewith, and tests made to ascertain that the products issued by manufacturers conform with the standards laid down. . . .

(e) That the method of control should include the licensing of manufacturers, inspection of their plant, premises and processes, and the testing of the finished products.

(f) That, with certain exceptions, testing by the Central Laboratory should be confined to samples taken from makers' stocks or bought in the open market, leaving to the manufacturers the primary responsibility for securing that the products conform with the prescribed standards and tests. That power should, however, be taken to require a manufacturer to submit for central testing, for a stated period, samples of every batch of a substance made.

(g) That power should be taken to inspect all premises where the substances are made and the several processes of their manufacture, but that in the case of Salvarsan and its analogues (Group B) and of the galenical and other preparations which we have classified as Group C, inspection should ordinarily be confined to the records and methods of biological testing and, when necessary, to the filling and sealing of the containers.

(h) That products made abroad should be subject to restrictions similar to those applying to products made in the United Kingdom and that licenses should be granted to approved manufacturers based upon a preliminary inspection of plant, premises and processes, and testing of samples. In addition, steps should be taken to ensure that each consignment attains the standards laid down for products of home manufacture. . . .

The report also included the outlines of a draft bill to implement the recommendations.[1]

The recommendations of the Committee on Control of Therapeutic Substances undoubtedly led to the Therapeutic Substances Act of 1925. This applied to vaccines, sera, toxins, antitoxins, antigens, arsphenamine and analogous substances, insulin, and posterior pituitary injection. The Act included most of the recommendations of the Committee, but the licensing authorities were the Health Ministers. Regulations issued between 1925 and 1956 brought catgut and other sutures, blood products, penicillin and some other antibiotics, tubocurarine and related products, and corticotrophin and corticosteroids under control. Standards were continuously kept under review and improved by a series of regulations. The Act was revised and consolidated in 1956. By new regulations made under this Act, absorbable hemostatics, enzymes used parenterally, and heparin were added. Therapeutic substances are thus adequately controlled.

1. Great Britain, Ministry of Health, Committee on Control of Certain Therapeutic Substances, *Report of the Departmental Committee Appointed to Consider and Advise upon the Legislative and Administrative Measures to Be Taken for the Effective Control of the Quality and Authenticity of Such Therapeutic Substances Offered for Sale to the Public as Cannot Be Tested Adequately by Direct Chemical Means* (London: H. M. Stationery Office, 1921).

The Food and Drugs Act of 1928

Three years after the passing of the Therapeutic Substances Act, a new Food and Drugs Act was passed, that of 1928. It repealed the whole of several earlier Acts and parts of others. Among the general provisions were:

> No person shall mix, colour, stain, or powder or order or permit any other person to mix, colour, stain, or powder . . . any drug with any ingredient or material so as to affect injuriously the quality or potency of the drug with the intent that the . . . drug may be sold in that state.
> No person shall sell any . . . drug so mixed, coloured, stained or powdered as aforesaid.
> . . . .
> No person shall sell to the prejudice of the purchaser . . . any drug which is not of the nature, or not of the substance, or not of the quality, of the article demanded by the purchaser.

The Act specified the local authorities responsible for administration of its provisions. These were the Common Council of the City of London, the metropolitan borough councils, and the county borough and county councils. These authorities have the duty to provide proper security for the sale of food and drugs in a pure and genuine condition and in particular to direct their officers to procure samples for analysis. If the Minister of Health, after communication with the Food and Drugs Authorities, is of the opinion that the authorities have failed to execute or enforce any of the provisions of the Act, he may empower any officer to execute and enforce them. Samples taken under the Act are submitted to public analysts for testing. The Act gave a limited right of entry of Ministry inspectors to certain food factories which had to be registered under the Act. This did not apply to drug manufacturers.

Samples of various relatively simple substances were taken from pharmacies under this and the earlier act, such as sugar of milk, sweet spirits of niter, camphorated oil, tincture of iodine, milk of sulphur, and effervescing citrate of magnesia. There were disputes about the results of some of the analyses of these products and about what the public actually desired when they asked for them. In 1924, therefore, a Joint Conference of the Pharmaceutical Society's Council, the Society of Public Analysts (later the Society for Analytical Chemistry), and the Retail Pharmacists' Union made some recommendations which were endorsed by the Ministry of Health. As a result a memorandum was sent to Public Health Authorities and this resolved some of the difficulties relating to sampling under the Food and Drugs Act.

It is obvious that the Food and Drugs Act was of very limited scope as far as drugs were concerned. In practice, a limited number of samples were taken, and these were usually restricted to rather simple substances which were easy to analyze.

The Pharmacy and Medicines Act of 1941

The provisions of this Act relating to the quality of drugs were the clauses restricting dispensing largely to pharmacies (except for rural dispensing practices) and requiring a declaration of the composition of all substances for which medicinal properties were claimed. This meant the end of the secret remedy and meant also that proprietary medicines could be analyzed to ensure that they complied with their declared formulae.

The Medicines Bill of 1968

In February, 1968, the Minister of Health introduced the Medicines Bill, which is at present (May, 1968) in the committee stage. New legislation has been contemplated for several years. The last Conservative Government issued a confidential memorandum outlining a proposed bill, and numerous organizations commented on this. The thalidomide tragedies undoubtedly hastened the introduction of the bill; after them, the Standing Medical Advisory Committees for England and Wales and Scotland set up a Joint Sub-Committee on Safety of Drugs with the following terms of reference:

> To advise the Minister of Health and the Secretary of State for Scotland on what measures are needed:—
> (i) to secure adequate pharmacological and safety testing and clinical trials of new drugs before their release for general use;
> (ii) to secure early detection of adverse effects arising after their release for general use; and
> (iii) to keep doctors informed of the experience of such drugs in clinical practice.

In an interim report of November, 1962, the Sub-Committee made the following recommendations:

(1) The responsibility for the experimental laboratory testing of new drugs before they are used in clinical trials should remain with the individual pharmaceutical manufacturer.
(2) It is neither desirable nor practicable that at this stage of their evaluation the responsibility for testing drugs should be transferred to a central authority.
(3) There should be an expert body to review the evidence and offer advice on the toxicity of new drugs, whether manufactured in Great Britain or abroad, before they are used in clinical trials. . . .

In their final report in 1963, the Sub-Committee further recommended that an expert body, to be known as the Committee on Safety of Drugs, should be set up with sub-committees to advise on (1) toxicity,

(2) clinical trials and therapeutic efficacy, and (3) adverse reactions. The six medical members recommended that the Committee should be set up in the first instance, pending legislation, on a voluntary basis, but that all new drugs and preparations should be submitted to it. The two pharmacist members issued a minority report pointing out the disadvantages of a voluntary scheme and calling for early comprehensive legislation to bring the whole field of drug safety and quality under the responsibility of the Health Ministers advised by a central body of experts.[2] The Committee was set up on a voluntary basis in 1963, and the pharmaceutical industry has collaborated with it very well.

In September, 1967, a White Paper was published outlining the proposal to be contained in the Medicines Bill,[3] and shortly afterward there appeared the *Report* of the Committee of Enquiry into the Relationship of the Pharmaceutical Industry with the National Health Service (the Sainsbury Report).[4] Both contained a proposal for the setting up of a Medicines Commission and for the requirement of a license before a drug or preparation can be marketed or imported. The Sainsbury Report recommended that the Medicines Commission should be independent, but the White Paper stated that it would be responsible to the Health Ministers, and this is included in the Bill. The Commission will have the duty of advising the Ministers on all aspects of safety, efficacy, and quality of drugs. It will advise on the setting up of committees, which will, however, be responsible to the Ministers. One of these will undoubtedly be equivalent to the Committee on Safety of Drugs.

Under the Bill, licenses will be required for the manufacture, importation, and marketing of all new drugs. Manufacturers will be required to show that their products are safe and efficacious. Certificates will be required before new drugs can be submitted for clinical trial. The licensing body will be the Health Ministers, and they will have the power to satisfy themselves as to the suitability of the premises and the qualifications of the staff of the manufacturers. They will have the right of inspection of premises and pharmacies and will be able to lay down systems of work and to check records. Eventually all preparations on the market will be brought under the licensing system.

2. Great Britain, Standing Medical Advisory Committees, Joint Sub-Committee on Safety of Drugs, *Safety of Drugs: Final Report* (London: H. M. Stationery Office, 1963).
3. *Forthcoming Legislation on the Safety, Quality and Description of Drugs and Medicines*, Presented to Parliament by the Secretary of State for Scotland, the Minister of Agriculture, Fisheries and Food, and the Minister of Health, September, 1967 (London: H. M. Stationery Office, 1967).
4. Great Britain, Committee of Enquiry into the Relationship of the Pharmaceutical Industry with the National Health Service (Chairman: Lord Sainsbury), *Report*, Presented to Parliament by the Minister of Health and the Secretary of State for Scotland, September, 1967 (London: H. M. Stationery Office, 1967).

The new Bill will take over the quality control requirements from the Food and Drugs Act and the Therapeutic Substances Act. Wholesalers will also be required to hold a licence and will be subject to inspection to ensure that their premises and facilities will guarantee the conservation of the activity of medicaments. Hygienic standards will be enforced for the manufacture, transportation, storage, and sale of all drugs. The British Pharmacopoeia Commission and its laboratories will be taken over by the Ministry of Health, which will have power to publish further formularies or compendia if this is thought necessary.

When it becomes law,* this Bill, which also contains many clauses about the legal control and sale of drugs, will give Great Britain its first really comprehensive legislation on medicines, and will give the public the best possible protection in the light of modern knowledge.

* Passed October 25, 1968.—Editor's Note.

Commentary

Melvin P. Earles

The preceding papers have raised some problems of definition regarding the title of this conference. I will not enter into a discussion on the definition of the term "drug," but I would point out that the subject has already extended into the wider field of drugs and their preparations. The British White Paper of 1967 observes that the use of the word "drug" to include both substance and preparation is confusing and, as we have seen, the subsequent legislation in Britain has been entitled the "Medicines Bill."

The principal feature of the three papers above has been control of purity, and each author has indicated the interlocking of social and scientific factors contributing to the standardization of the quality of medicines and the elimination of adulteration. As the conference proceeds we will see that a complex of social pressures and scientific advances contributes in a similar manner to other problems of drug control, in particular control of efficacy and safety.

It has been clearly indicated that success in control of quality of drugs is dependent upon the establishment and acceptance of satisfactory standards. One result has been that over the period under discussion, as scientific methods have advanced, the pharmacopoeias have been transformed from formularies ensuring uniformity of preparations to books of standards. The papers have described the process in respect to drug purity. I would like to indicate some of the problems involved when we consider the pharmacopoeias as controlling factors in a context wider than that of drug purity.

A major development in the history of therapeutics in the early nineteenth century was the introduction of some new and highly active remedies, notably the alkaloids and hydrocyanic acid. The latter, a highly toxic substance, introduces us to a major problem associated with the concept of an "official" pharmacopoeia. François Magendie's "Mémoire sur l'emploi de l'acide prussique dans le traitement de plusieurs maladies de poitrine, et particulièrement dans la phthisie pulmonaire" was published in *Annales de chimie et de physique* in 1817. The paper was published in an English translation in the *Journal of Science* by A. B. Granville in 1818 and again brought to the attention of British physicians by translations of Magendie's *Formulaire pour la préparation et l'emploi de*

38

nouveaux médicamens of 1821. The records of the sale of hydrocyanic acid in London about this time suggest that it was being extensively used not only for pulmonary conditions, as recommended by Magendie, but also as a sedative, after John Elliotson's discovery in about 1820 of its sedative effect in cases of gastrodynia.

Diluted hydrocyanic acid was included in an appendix to the French *Codex medicamentarius* of 1818 and included in the first *United States Pharmacopoeia* of 1820. The compilers of the *Pharmacopoeia Londinensis*, however, hesitated, and did not include it in the 1824 edition. Their opposition rested upon its extreme toxicity and doubtful therapeutic value. Thomas Cox, discussing the matter in his translation of the London pharmacopoeia of 1824, observed that "something further must be known before we prescribe it." Nevertheless, at the time it was being extensively prescribed, and, with such a highly active material with a strength dependent upon mode of preparation, it would have been in the interests of safety to follow the example of the French and the Americans and insert a monograph in the London pharmacopoeia. On the other hand, to have included it would have bestowed upon hydrocyanic acid the accolade of therapeutic efficiency. This might be considered an early example of the delay between the introduction and use in therapy of a potentially hazardous substance and the appearance of pharmacopoeial data controlling strength and dose. This particular delay ended with the next edition of the pharmacopoeia in 1836. Until that time the shortcomings of the pharmacopoeia were compensated by commentaries such as S. F. Gray's *A Treatise on Pharmacology*. In the third edition of that work (1824), in his discussion of prussic acid, Gray commented that one should not wait for a new edition of the pharmacopoeia to regulate the strength and preparations of new drugs.

Hydrocyanic acid was introduced into medicine at a time when judgment in therapeutics relied upon the habits, observations, and prejudices of clinical experience. It is an interesting fact that in his memoir on this substance Magendie predicted the use of animal experiments to determine the mode of action of medicaments "so that it becomes easier to vary their effects and to remedy their disadvantages." Many years were to elapse, however, before advances in physiology and chemistry permitted a fruitful exploitation of physiological experiment for the progress of pharmacodynamic knowledge and the advance of therapeutics. Meanwhile, as we have seen from the papers under discussion, the major developments were devoted to improvement of drug purity.

An examination of the British pharmacopoeias of 1914 and 1932 will unquestionably support the history of progress in drug standardization as outlined by Dr. Whittet. On close inspection, however, there appears to be a preoccupation with purity of drugs and some neglect of other matters, notably the control of efficacy of the preparations. I would illustrate this by referring to the example of compressed tablets.

A patent for a machine to compress medicinal substances was issued to William Brockendon in 1843, and thereafter there was a steady increase in the marketing of compressed drugs, which were offered as an alternative to pills. Correspondence in the *Chemist and Druggist* in 1881 indicates that compressing machines were in demand, and in 1903 the firm of Allen and Hanburys introduced the prototype of the modern high-output rotary machine. The technology of tablet-making is sufficient to indicate the extensive use of this convenient form of medication by the turn of the century. The *British Pharmacopoeia* of 1914, however, refers to only one tablet. This was *Tabella Glycerylis Trinitratis*, a product which differed from other tablets in that it was intended to be chewed, not swallowed. There was no change in the pharmacopoeia of 1932.

The efficacy of a compressed tablet is dependent upon a number of factors. First, the medicament must be uniformly mixed with the base, to ensure the proper dose in each tablet. Second, there must be a uniformity of weight throughout the batch. Finally, the rate of disintegration in the stomach will determine the release of the active ingredient and its absorption. In Britain, tests to control these variations were not official until 1945, when tablet monographs were eventually admitted to the pharmacopoeia in the seventh addendum to the *B.P.* of 1932. Until that time the only contribution of the pharmacopoeia to tablet control had been to ensure that the active constituent conformed to standards of purity. The advantage of purity, however, was lost if, as a result of inadequate mixing, the unit tablet was deficient in weight of active ingredient, or if, because of machine variation, the weights of the tablets varied throughout the batch. Furthermore, there is little advantage in enclosing a pure drug in a tablet which, because of overcompression or poor formulation, passes through the body without disintegrating!

Whatever the reason for the delay, the fact remains that both the *British Pharmacopoeia* and the *United States Pharmacopoeia* failed for many years to control a preparation in common use. With more recent advances in pharmaceutical technology and the appearance of new unit dosage forms, the situation has been repeated.

The pharmacopoeia has been shown to be a useful instrument in the development of standards to control drug purity. Has it been of equal value in the control of wider problems arising from the rapid advances in drug therapy? How much truth is there in the statement by Wyndham Davies in his book *The Pharmaceutical Industry* (1967)? "Long term thinking may eventually lead to the admission that although there may always need to be some kind of a list of official remedies, the pharmacopoeia as known today is virtually obsolete."

Commentary

Gert Brieger

In commenting upon these three interesting papers dealing with the European backgrounds of the history of drug control, particularly in France and England, I should like to confine my few remarks to some general points.

I would like to approach these papers from the point of view of a medical historian. As a medical historian, I am, of course, very much interested in the relationship of drug control to the practice of medicine at any given time. In the nineteenth century, for instance, there was probably a fairly widespread feeling among people in both Europe and America that some sort of protection or control ought to exist. Both Dr. Stieb and Dr. Berman cited specific ways in which this was attempted or carried out. I believe, however, that we know too little of what actually was going on at the practitioners' level. There is a need, it seems to me, for much more study of the roles of the physicians and of their patients in the endeavor to protect the public from false claims, from impure drugs, and from badly prescribed or poorly administered remedies.

The papers have given us a wealth of information in regard to the problems of control, both legislative and professionally exerted. We have not heard, nor do we usually seem to hear much, of the problems of drug control in the practice of medicine. In defense of the authors, I hasten to add that this was not their intention. I do not wish to criticize them for what they have not set out to do, for they deserve praise for what they did accomplish.

I would like to echo the sentiments of Professor Ackerknecht, who recently wrote the following: "Since our contemporaries in consultative practice are well aware of the gap which even now exists between the medicine preached and the medicine generally practised, and since studies are available which reveal the width of this gap in the 20th century, it is time that historians looked hard at the actualities of the past." These lines come from a short article that Professor Ackerknecht called "A Plea for a 'Behaviorist' Approach in Writing the History of Medicine."[1] I think that the subject of drug control is also deserving of a behaviorist approach.

1. *J. Hist. Med.* 22 (1967): 211–14.

Certainly we must know the legislative history of drug control, but we must also learn more about the actual conditions of prescribing the drugs and delivering them to the patients. That the physician prescribed a drug which he had every expectation of being given to the patient in the proper form, but that in fact the patient was poisoned as a result, was a fairly common occurrence, at least in this country and probably in Europe as well. For example, the pharmacist in America might have been unable to read a nearly illegible prescription written on a scrap of newspaper or the edge of a napkin. One medical editor in this country suggested in 1864 that the name of the patient ought to be required on each prescription, so that there would be less chance for children to be given doses actually prescribed for their parents. This was apparently already a requirement in Germany at the time. This particular medical editor, who was writing from New York, had many things to say about prescription writing, for example:

> There is another particular in which physicians are even more reprehensible, for it is the result of gross carelessness. There are many physicians in this city in large practice who rarely write the directions on prescriptions, or even the doses. The directions are given to the friends at home, who in their grief or excitement frequently forget what is said, and as the druggist cannot enlighten them, the medicines are very likely improperly administered.[2]

This is only one of many possible examples. These problems are part of the broader history of therapeutics, it is true, but they belong to the story of drug control as well.

As Dr. Berman has mentioned, there were many parallels between French methods of solving the problem of drug control and those of other countries. Many of the issues and the responses were encountered in this country as well as in Britain and France. None of the participants, however, addressed himself to the conditions on the rest of the European continent, outside of France. Nor am I going to undertake that task.

Not only must one view the problem of drug control as an important and interesting facet of governmental and professional interaction, but one must also consider the place of several other institutions, some of which have been discussed above. Specifically, I would include the press, both newspapers and medical journals, the schools of medicine and pharmacy, the medical and scientific societies, and, in the United States at least, the religious organizations and their newspapers. All these certainly played a part in the final regulation of just what drug was prescribed by physicians and pseudo-physicians and given to the patient— who, after all, was the main beneficiary of the regulations we have been discussing.

2. [Stephen Smith], "Prescription Writing," *Amer. Med. Times* 8 (1864): 262–63.

Discussion

Dr. Blake: Our first commentator addressed a specific question to Dr. Whittet; would you like to comment on it?

Dr. Whittet: Dr. Earles has raised a very important point, and I agree with him entirely that the pharmacopoeia has changed in character from a book of formulae to a book of standards. I think that it is now in yet another transitional stage. I hope pharmacopoeias will not disappear. I think there will be a continuing need for standards.

It is very important, indeed, that we get agreement on standards. I know from my experience on the European Pharmacopoeia Commission what a difficult task this is. We hope to publish the first volume this year, and at the moment we have touched only such things as sodium chloride. We hope to get to the more advanced ones in the second volume. We all said, "Sodium chloride is a nice easy one; there will be no trouble about this." Then we found that nearly every country puts in a different substance to stop caking, and I have seen a whole morning's debate on just this.

The point that Professor Earles raised about availability is also very important. I have been interested in this for a long time, and I know that Dr. Francke has been also. I remember one of his early articles pointing out that, however good a drug is, unless it is properly absorbed, it is useless. I had an example of this myself with cortisone. When I was at University College Hospital, cortisone was offered by some Italian manufacturers at about a quarter, or even less, of the price in Britain. I hesitated about getting it for a long time because I was doubtful about its quality. Eventually I felt that I had to tell my drug and therapeutics committee that I could buy it at a much cheaper rate but that I was not entirely satisfied about it, and they left it to me to do what I thought appropriate. The London Teaching Hospitals Joint Contracting Committee then bought samples from the firm—in such a way that the firm did not know where they were going—and had them tested. They complied with the *British Pharmacopoeia* in every way. Finally I bought some for use in my hospital, and within a week or so eleven patients who had been very well stabilized for Addison's disease on cortisone went into Addisonian crisis. We immediately impounded the tablets and had them assayed, and, again, they complied completely with the requirements of the *Pharmacopoeia*. When I looked at them under the microscope, however, the faulty tablets had enormous aggregates; obviously they were not being absorbed. Of course, this is well known now: this was one of the very early examples. There are many others. I think it is important that we look at therapeutic availability, and I was pleased to learn yesterday that the United States Pharmacopeial Convention has set up a committee for this purpose.

My own view is that pharmacopoeias will continue, and that they should continue. I think I would like to see them in looseleaf form, like the Belgian one, so that one can insert revisions immediately. While I am sure they should continue, unless they keep up to date in regard to availability, they will become obsolete.

Dr. Cooper: I am rather interested in the last remarks about the future role of pharmacopoeias. If we could dissociate ourselves from the format problem, I doubt whether many would disagree that we need a master compendium of information. But does the dispensing pharmacist any longer require this very expensive work, which in this country is called the *Pharmacopeia of the United States* or perhaps the *National Formulary*? I have asked some number of pharmacists what they use it for. So far as I can discern, in this age of manufactured preparations they mostly bring it over to the lunch counter for small children to sit on. Yet by law, in most of our states, they must have it on hand; it ranks somewhat with the bottle of colored water. The question is, who needs this pharmacopoeia? This is an economic problem. It relates to the question of format, which Dr. Whittet mentioned. Should it be looseleaf, or should it perhaps be an electronic compendium of all that is known about drugs and preparations from which one could draw information selectively?

Dr. Whittet: It is quite true that the *Pharmacopoeia* is of very slight use to the general practitioner in pharmacy, and we find in Britain that the volume known as the *Extra Pharmacopoeia*, or Martindale, really contains all that he wants. I know that some pharmacies do not have the *Pharmacopoeia* at all.

Dr. Young: There was a paper which is perhaps pertinent to this point given at the American Pharmaceutical Association meeting last week by a young behavioral scientist from the Ohio State University School of Pharmacy, as I recall—a paper which is also related to Dr. Brieger's questions about how the art is practiced—in which he investigated how much use pharmacists make of data like the *Pharmacopeia* or new drug brochures. This was an experiment using thirty-six pharmacists, presumably in the region of Columbus, in which various questions were posed to them, first over the telephone by persons assuming the role of a physician, and second by students who came in with prescriptions as if they were patients, to see how well the pharmacists applied the knowledge that they should have. I do not remember the exact details except in one illustrative case in which one individual got two prescriptions filled a week apart. Although brochures on both of these drugs used the most stirring language that the Food and Drug Administration presumably could get the manufacturers to employ in warning that simultaneous use of these drugs was absolutely contraindicated, only one of the thirty-six druggists, as I recall, pointed out to the purchaser the risk he was running by using these two drugs simultaneously. This may have been the most egregious case, but in every instance, I think, if you use 60 per cent as flunking, the pharmacists in this experiment flunked. So, it seems to me this study relates both to Dr. Cooper's question about the use of these works by pharmacists and doctors and to Dr. Brieger's point about studying how pharmacy, or medicine, is really practiced.

Dr. Stieb: The question of therapeutic efficacy, I think, is one that we have really become seriously concerned about only within the last decade. It has come primarily because of the growing concern of governments everywhere with the cost of drugs and with generic prescribing. This immediately raises the question of whether drugs the same in formula are really the same in effect.

Dr. Francke: I would like to comment about the use of the *Pharmacopeia* by the practicing pharmacist and to point out how the entrance of the government into the medical care picture has brought about the need for testing drugs for physiological availability. In the hospital the pharmacist needs a pharmacopoeia in order to prepare specifications for the quality of drugs to be purchased, because traditionally the hospital pharmacist has purchased drugs under generic names. From the pharmaceutical industry's point of view this seems a very poor system, but the industry loses sight of one important aspect of the hospital pharmacist's purchases, and that is his control of the source of supply. If he is purchasing a drug like cortisone, he selects the major sources of supply, sends bids to all of them, and obtains a very good product at a very low price. With the entrance of the government more fully into medical care, the general public has discovered that hospitals have been obtaining these low prices, and it wants all drugs purchased and dispensed generically. However, unless the source of supply is controlled, the purchase of drugs under their generic or nonproprietary name can be dangerous. This is shown by the experience of the Department of Defense.

The Department of Defense, which procures all the drugs for the government, sends out inspectors to inspect pharmaceutical plants which wish to submit bids for government business. Fifty per cent of the plants inspected are turned down because their products do not meet the specifications. Yet all these products are labeled *"USP"* or *"NF,"* they are on the American market, and where they go we do not know. This is an important bottleneck in the control of drugs in the United States.

Because of this situation, people are now saying—even the *USP* and the *NF* have now said—that we can no longer be satisfied with the *USP* label or assume that a drug which meets the specifications of the *USP* will be automatically acceptable. It has to be proved physiologically available and therapeutically effective.

Dr. Ackerknecht: I believe that the question of psychology came up in another connection. If you hear the paper of Professor Berman and then add to it some personal experience in French pharmacies, the old French proverb, *plus ça change, plus c'est la même chose*—the more it changes, the more it's the same thing—comes to mind. I go very often to France, and each time I am simply flabbergasted by the number of proprietary medicines intentionally made to look old-fashioned which are handed out there. This brings me to a psychological problem. There are two equally irrational attitudes toward drugs: the one, this is an old drug and that is very good, and the other, this is a new drug, this is excellent. These two attitudes seem to be differently distributed in several countries. In France, the number of people who still believe that an old drug must be good seems to be larger. But I think it would be very enlightening if we could get a little bit closer to the basic attitudes behind these views of old and new drugs.

I think also it would be not so bad to look a little bit at the very close connection between politics and drug control. Perhaps it is so self-evident that nobody mentions it, but it is really no accident that it was in the beginning of the twentieth century that the law-givers were very much stimulated to do something in this direction.

There is another point which might be perhaps disliked. There is, especially in small towns, a certain tender relationship between the apothecary and the doctors, and I think that this has had a tremendous influence on drug control. I mean, of course, the economic relationship. If you want an illustration, which is, of course, purely fictitious, take Dr. Knock, created by Jules Romains—but I have seen similar things in life. This is a fact that is not often mentioned except in the codes of ethics of the medical profession. That is one of the first things doctors are warned not to do. It is not impossible that things like this tender relationship might have had something to do with why drug control in some quarters did not develop so fast.

Dr. Berman: The psychological element is very important. I did not have time or space to elaborate upon it, but certainly theriac is a wonderful example which in France goes right back to Moïse Charas in the seventeenth century, and even earlier. Later, in the nineteenth century, when Trousseau, Bouchardat, and others refer to theriac as chaotic and bizarre, they display an ambivalent attitude. They cannot rid themselves of this attitude: theriac is a monster, but it is a monster which they love. The tradition and the psychological element are extremely significant.

Part II: Scientific Backgrounds

A Short Survey of Drug Therapy Prior to 1900

Erwin H. Ackerknecht

Drug therapy is generally linked with certain theories. But it is very often hard to say whether these theories are actually the guideposts of the respective treatments or rationalizations justifying the use of much older methods and materials, as Temkin has shown, for example, in the case of the Galenic use of cathartics.[1] Whether guidepost or rationalization, these theories are, in any case, markers indicating the presence of certain therapeutic practices and can be used as such in a reconstruction of the therapeutic past. In such a reconstruction we have to be careful not to overlook those therapeutic measures that were used without theory.

In primitive medicine, where the cause of disease and the action of a drug were considered magic, there was little place for trial and error and even less for experiment to ascertain the effects of drugs.[2] In Egyptian medicine, the prototype of archaic medicine and a mixture of magic and naturalistic procedures, drug therapy was predominant, and, for as long as we have written prescriptions, we have used the Egyptian formula as a model. Surprisingly enough, we find no venesection and almost no diet mentioned in the papyri. As we know very little about Egyptian ideas underlying drug treatments and nothing about Egyptian methods of assessing their value, a discussion of Egyptian drugs seems not very relevant to our problem.

Greek medicine, however, was no longer based on supernaturalism. The magic implication of the expression *pharmakon* seems to have disappeared during the seventh century B.C.[3] The Hippocratic physician (fourth century B.C.) treated the state of the sick individual, not the disease. He tried to support "nature," which acted through coction of the humors. Diet in its largest sense (comprising also exercise, baths, and psychological influences) and evacuation by purgatives were the main instruments of the physician. Other drugs were used occasionally, mostly in surgical salves.

---

1. O. Temkin, "Historical Aspects of Drug Therapy," in Paul Talalay, ed., *Drugs in Our Society* (Baltimore: Johns Hopkins Press, 1964), p. 4. See also E. H. Ackerknecht, "Aspects of the History of Therapeutics," *Bull. Hist. Med.* 36 (1962): 389–419.

2. E. H. Ackerknecht, "Natural Diseases and Rational Treatment in Primitive Medicine," *Bull. Hist. Med.* 19 (1946): 467–97.

3. Walter Artelt, *Studien zur Geschichte der Begriffe "Heilmittel" und "Gift,"* Studien zur Geschichte der Medizin, no. 23 (Leipzig: J. A. Barth, 1937), p. 47.

In Alexandrian medicine (third century B.C.) the use of bleeding and drugs increased tremendously. The great reformer Asclepiades (born 124 B.C.), the first prominent Greek physician in Rome, reversed this trend for a while by reducing the use of drugs, venesection, and purgatives and by recommending diet and water.

Galen (130–201 A.D.), whose synthesis of Greek medicine ruled medicine for over 1,300 years, claimed to be a follower of Hippocrates. Actually, he was a dogmatic rationalist, recommending the extensive use of bleeding, purging, and drugs, often in the particularly undesirable form of mixed drugs like his notorious theriac. The uncritical polypharmacy of late Greek medicine was also reflected in the materia medica of Dioscorides (ca. 50 A.D.), which contains almost three times the number of medicinal plants mentioned in the Hippocratic writings.

Medieval medicine in both the East and the West was mostly Galenic. The Arabs added a number of Eastern drugs and began the use of metal remedies.[4]

With Paracelsus, the great Renaissance revolutionary, chemistry— still called alchemy—entered medicine for good, providing new theories of disease as well as new medicaments. Galenic plant drugs were often replaced by laboratory-produced mineral drugs. Paracelsus drove out specific diseases with specifics, called arcana. He and his followers claimed that experience was more valuable than tradition. During the Renaissance potent exotic drugs, such as guaiac and tobacco, were first used; however, some of the most important ones—Peruvian bark, ipecacuanha—did not arrive until the seventeenth century.

Under these influences the old Galenic system of therapy began to disintegrate. The traditional methods of derivation and revulsion were mixed with or replaced by new ones. A chaos of opinions and practices came into being which culminated and ended only in the nineteenth century. Hippocratic expectation regained some support.

Seventeenth-century therapeutics were very strongly influenced by iatrochemists such as van Helmont and Sylvius who did not practice bloodletting. Zimmermann called them mere apothecaries. All their chemically prepared mineral drugs had the great advantage of remaining nearly identical in their effects, as compared to drugs taken from the plant and animal kingdoms. With the seventeenth-century traditionalists, bleeding and purging reached unheard-of proportions. Sydenham is usually praised as an empiricist, which he certainly was in his use of Peruvian bark, but in general his practice was far more aprioristic than is usually recognized.

    4. S. Hamarneh, "Climax of Chemical Therapy in 10th Century Arabic Medicine," *Der Islam* 38 (1963): 283ff.

In the eighteenth century expectation, which implies the existence of a certain therapeutic skepticism, was recommended by such diverse clinicians as Boerhaave, Stahl, F. Hoffmann, Tronchin, and Heberden. The incorporation of numerous folk remedies, including digitalis, belladonna, cod-liver oil, ergot, and vaccination, was also significant. Yet tradition prevailed with bleeding, purging, and vomiting, and the incredible abuse of toxic substances like antimony and mercury.

This traditionalistic eclecticism lasted into the second half of the nineteenth century.[5] The three early reform movements, Brunonianism, Broussaisism, and Rasorism, were worse than the evils they were supposed to cure. Relief was first brought by the "skepticism" of the Paris and Vienna schools. The public expressed its opinion by sponsoring sects like the Thomsonians, the homeopaths, and the "water doctors."

The way out was "physiologism." Magendie, father of experimental physiology, experimental pathology, and experimental pharmacology, transformed traditional materia medica into experimental pharmacology. His *Formulaire*, which discussed the therapeutic use of the newly discovered alkaloids and halogens on the basis of animal experimentation, appeared for the first time in 1821. But progress was slow, and the "antipyretic wave" of the second half of the century shows that physiologism too could go wrong. One of its successes was hormone treatment (Brown-Séquard, 1889, and Murray, 1891). The triumph of physiologism and the beginning of a new era in therapeutics were heralded by the antisera of Behring, after 1890, and the chemotherapy of Ehrlich, after 1904.

Evaluation of Drugs

Asked how they would evaluate the effect of their drugs, most ancient physicians would probably have answered: through experience with different patients. New drugs were tried out the same way. There were, of course, also rationalists or dogmatics who frankly judged a drug primarily in relation to its consistency with a given theory of disease. However, if we examine the actual practice of all physicians objectively, we must come to the following conclusion: some rationalism but, *above all, tradition and the opinion of the profession* have always very heavily influenced the practice of even those physicians who thought themselves to be pure empiricists. J. G. Zimmermann rightly stated in 1761 that the "experience" of most physicians was but "pseudo experience."[6] This

5. For their survival in American therapeutics, see Alex Berman, "The Heroic Approach in 19th Century Therapeutics," *Bull. Amer. Soc. Hosp. Pharm.* 11 (1954): 321–27.

6. J. G. Zimmermann, *Von der Erfahrung in der Arzneykunst*, 3d ed. (Zurich: Orell, Füssli, 1831), pp. 3ff.

was almost unavoidable, as methods to evaluate the effect of drugs successfully and to objectivate experience developed very slowly.

Apparently the first to look systematically for methods of organizing
therapeutic experience in such a way that valid results could be obtained
were the members of the Alexandrian medical sect of the third century
B.C. who called themselves empiricists.[7] Their practice centered around
the use of drugs. Like all empirical rebellions, theirs ran into a dead end.[8]
Their most valuable insights—the necessity of repeating experiences and
of noting negative instances—were forgotten.

Galen is rightly famous as an experimentalist in physiology. He
occasionally reported therapeutic observations ("experiments") or self-
experiments. But he was a violent critic of the empiricists. Theoretically,
he tried to balance reason and experience. Practically, his legacy in
therapeutics was dogmatism. As Zimmermann says: "He taught us to
reason so well on the basis of wrong premises."[9] The same is true of
the medieval Arabs: they performed a few experiments, but dogmatism
was the dominant method in their therapeutics.

In the sixteenth century greater emphasis on experience was observ-
able as a complement to the beginning decline of traditionalist Aristo-
telianism and Galenism and to the influx of new exotic drugs. Paré
reported the use of controls in a therapeutic experiment.[10] Gesner undertook numerous self-experiments with drugs,[11] and certain attempts at clinical empiricism were made by physicians, especially in treating syphilis and
in using new drugs. But a "philosophy of medical experience" was still
lacking. Paracelsus the alchemist was familiar with experiments, but
Paracelsus the mystic despised such lowly ways of finding out whether
something worked. His *experientia* meant exploring the drug through
mystical communion—something close to religious experience.[12]

With Francis Bacon (whose *Novum organum* appeared in 1620) began
the long lineage of the modern philosophers of experience. But it is a long
way from a philosophy of experience to effectively organized experience.
Bacon wanted to apply his method of induction to medicine. He favored
experimentation, though he called contemporary experiments—probably
aiming at the alchemists—"blind and stupid." He rediscovered the necessity of repeated experience and of reporting negative facts. His own

7. Karl Deichgräber, *Die griechische Empirikerschule* (Berlin: Weidmann, 1930).
8. E. H. Ackerknecht, "Recurrent Themes in Medical Thought," *Sci. Monthly*
69 (1949): 80–83.
9. Zimmermann, *Von der Erfahrung*, p. 27.
10. H. E. Sigerist, "Ambroise Paré's Onion Treatment of Burns," *Bull. Hist.
Med.* 15 (1944): 143–49.
11. Hans Fischer, *Conrad Gessner . . .: Leben und Werk*, Veröffentlichung der
Naturforschenden Gesellschaft in Zürich (Zurich: Leemann, 1966), pp. 80–81.
12. Paracelsus, *Sämtliche Werke*, ed. Karl Sudhoff (Munich: R. Oldenbourg,
1922–33), 10: 284–87; Walter Pagel, *Paracelsus* (Basel: S. Karger, 1958), p. 51.

application of his method yielded no valuable results, however. Baglivi, who was strongly influenced by Bacon, had nothing new to say. Actually, in his devotion to the ancients, he was even less progressive than Bacon.[13]

Sennert's promising chapter, "De modo investigandis vires medicamentorum," gave but a few rules: experience is more important than reasoning; *repeated* observations *in man* of *one* medicament in *simple* diseases are necessary.[14] I have found no indications that he actually practiced his precepts.

The seventeenth century was a century of animal experimentation. Harvey was by no means exceptional in this respect, although the success of his experiments was exceptional. Most experimentalists of the seventeenth century were less lucky: intravenous medication, for example, was found experimentally but had to be abandoned.[15] Still, Wepfer's toxicological experiments in animals could have served as a model to future generations.[16] Willis' excellent animal experiments with drugs were inexplicably forgotten.[17] Van Helmont's experiments upon himself were without consequence.[18] The excellent observer and friend of Locke, Sydenham, who compared physicians to cooks,[19] certainly tried, sometimes successfully, to be an empiricist in therapeutics. Yet closer scrutiny shows that he depended on authority and dogma in most of his therapeutic actions. More therapeutics were based on actual clinical experience in the seventeenth century; a theory of experience and animal experimentation in therapeutics began to develop, but these phenomena remained peripheral.

The eighteenth century began to come to grips with the problem of drug evaluation, less through theory than through action. J. G. Zimmermann's work *On Experience* was very widely read for a long time (Claude Bernard quoted him). His criticism was often astute; for example, he showed that what is called experience is mostly *routine*. He reflected the reaction of the Enlightenment against the fossilized pseudo experience of craftsmen, and against "experiences" which actually were superstitions. But his sterile bookishness was not improved by his pre-romantic theory

13. Giorgio Baglivi, *Opera omnia medico-practica, et anatomica*, 9th ed. (Antwerp: J. F. Rüdiger, 1719), pp. 8ff.
14. Daniel Sennert, *Institutionum medicinae libri V* (Wittenberg: Heirs of T. Mevius, 1644), pp. 970ff.
15. Heinrich Buess, *Die historischen Grundlagen der intravenösen Injektion*, Veröffentlichungen der Schweizerischen Gesellschaft für Geschichte der Medizin und der Naturwissenschaften, no. 15 (Aarau: H. R. Sauerländer, 1946).
16. Hans Fischer, *Johann Jakob Wepfer, 1620–1695* (Zurich: A. Rudolf, 1931).
17. Thomas Willis, *Pharmaceutice rationalis*, pt. 1 (Oxford, 1674), pp. 54, 307. See also Hansruedi Isler, *Thomas Willis: Ein Wegbereiter der modernen Medizin, 1621–1675*, Grosse Naturforscher, vol. 29 (Stuttgart: Wissenschaftliche Verlagsgesellschaft, 1965), pp. 141ff.
18. J. B. van Helmont, *Ortus medicinae* (Amsterdam: L. Elzevir, 1652).
19. Kenneth Dewhurst, *John Locke (1632–1704), Physician and Philosopher* (London: Wellcome Historical Medical Library, 1963), p. 39.

that experience was a matter of "genius." It is amazing how little Zimmermann, who did so many animal experiments for Haller, has to say on this subject.

Withering's 1785 book on digitalis, with his 163 case histories, showed that mere simple clinical trial can give excellent results in the hands of a critical observer. The controlled clinical trial gained stature when James Lind, on May 20, 1747, treated twelve patients with scurvy by six different methods and proved the superiority of using citrus fruit.[20] The expression "placebo" began to enter medical language in the eighteenth century, but the use of placebos in clinical trials, though recommended earlier,[21] belongs to the twentieth.[22] Smallpox inoculation and vaccination were accompanied by numerous clinical trials, for example, those by Sloane, Jenner, and J. P. Frank. In 1873, however, Fonssagrives[23] still did not mention controls when discussing *l'expérimentation clinique!*

Melvin P. Earles has recently drawn attention to the early large-scale animal experiments of Langrish in 1746 with cherry-laurel water, which prepared the introduction (by Brera in 1809, and others) of hydrocyanic acid into therapy, and to those of Fontana on opium, which were part of the extensive experimentation with the drug (by Haller, Whytt, Monod, and others) in the second half of the eighteenth century. Both Langrish and Fontana, although they have not received much attention, showed great insight into the problems of therapeutic experimentation.[24] This cannot be said, however, of the eighteenth-century experimental work summarized by P. Bernkopf in his Berlin thesis of 1936.[25] Most of it was toxicological (Sproegel, 1753, and Hillefeld, 1760). Numerous substances were tested, but each one only once in one animal. This was also true in the case of such a distinguished experimentalist as Stephen Hales, who was also handicapped by his prejudices in favor of iatromechanical theory.

M. Lindenberger offered evidence in his Berlin thesis of 1937[26] for no less than seventeen authors of the eighteenth century who experimented with drugs on blood in vitro. Unfortunately, their premise that

20. James Lind, *A Treatise on the Scurvy*, 2d ed. (London: A. Millar, 1757), pp. 149ff.
21. O. Rosenbach, *Grundlagen, Aufgaben und Grenzen der Therapie* (Vienna, Leipzig: Urban & Schwarzenberg, 1891), p. 110.
22. P. Kissel and D. Barrucand, *Placebos et effet placebo en médecine* (Paris: Masson, 1964).
23. J. B. Fonssagrives, "Médicament," in *Dictionnaire encyclopédique des sciences médicales*, ed. A. Dechambre (Paris: G. Masson, P. Asselin, 1864–89), 2d ser., 6: 245ff.
24. M. P. Earles, "Experiments with Drugs and Poisons in the 17th and 18th Centuries," *Ann. Sci.* 19 (1963): 245–54; Earles, "The Introduction of Hydrocyanic Acid into Medicine," *Med. Hist.* 11 (1967): 305–13.
25. Pawel Bernkopf, *Tierversuche mit Arzneimitteln im 18. Jahrhundert*, inaugural dissertation (Berlin: L. Begach, 1936).
26. Manfred Lindenberger, *Pharmakologische Versuche mit dem menschlichen Blut in 18. Jahrhundert*, inaugural dissertation (Berlin: A. Tausk, 1937).

the effect in vivo and in vitro is identical was wrong. Otherwise, the work of some of them, like John Freind (1675–1728), who also made a few pharmaceutical experiments, and J. T. Eller (1689–1760), represented progress in experimental technique through the great number of experiments accomplished and the thoroughness with which they were undertaken.

Although Withering demonstrated that despite a poor method excellent results can be obtained by a critical observer, the work of A. Stoerck, the famous Vienna clinician, proves that with enthusiasts an apparently good method can produce pitiful errors. Looking for drugs against cancer and melancholy, he began in 1760 to test old and abandoned remedies like hemlock, datura, hyoscyamus, aconitum, and stramonium with an apparently irreproachable method. He tried the drugs first in animals, then in himself, and then submitted them to clinical trial. He reported tremendous and purely imaginary successes, using far too few cases, interpreting every positive result as being due to the drug, every negative one as due to "accident." No wonder that his disciple Hahnemann achieved, through experiments on himself, even stranger results.

Controlled clinical trials and pharmacological experimentation grew up in the eighteenth century, but they did not affect the most widely read authors on materia medica like Cullen and Arnemann. The breakthrough came in the early nineteenth century, when, also, the philosophy of experience culminated in the work of John Stuart Mill.

It is well known that the real founder of experimental pharmacology was François Magendie, who was followed by Claude Bernard, Buchheim, and others. Their work became possible only through the contemporary achievements of the apothecary-chemists who, for the first time, put pure, chemically identifiable, nonmineral substances like urea, the alkaloids, and the halogens into the hands of the experimenters. Progress was, of course, slow. Barbier, a great authority on therapeutics, was still repeating in 1819 the Linnean dictum that substances which do not smell or taste are pharmacologically inactive.[27]

The most rational form of the controlled clinical trial is due to the Paris School, and especially to P. C. A. Louis and the "numerical method" he introduced in the 1820's. Pinel, Esquirol, G. Bayle, Rostan, Laënnec, and others used therapeutic statistics before Louis, and Gavarret corrected his mathematics.[28] But with Louis, controlled clinical trials became routine. They were particularly frequent in the 1830's in relation to typhoid fever, pneumonia, and venesection.[29] The statistics of Louis, Marshall Hall,

27. J. B. G. Barbier, "Médicament," in *Dictionaire des sciences médicales* (Paris: C. L. F. Panckoucke, 1812–22), 32: 113.

28. E. H. Ackerknecht, *Medicine at the Paris Hospital, 1794–1848* (Baltimore: Johns Hopkins Press, 1967), pp. 9, 102–4.

29. R. H. Brochin, "Expectation," in *Dictionnaire*, ed. Dechambre, 1st ser., 36: 436–37.

and Dietl were to bring about the abandonment of this ancient panacea. I would not call the astute comparative observations of Semmelweis and Lister clinical trials, as is sometimes done. Clinical trials, by the way, were condemned by many—Wunderlich, for example[30]—as unethical.

It should not be forgotten that the two methods discussed above, statistical clinical trial and animal experimentation, were paralleled by a long line of self-experimentation, by investigators from Purkyne through the anesthetists, bacteriologists, and endocrinologists, to A. Hofmann and LSD.[31]

In spite of this tremendous progress during the nineteenth century in finding methods to evaluate therapeutic experience, Politzer in 1876 was still able to prepare a long list of therapeutic "sins" which were the result of insufficient evaluation.[32] And I wonder whether such a list could not be composed even today.

30. C. A. Wunderlich, "Ein Plan zur festeren Begründung der therapeutischen Erfahrungen," *Schmidt's Jahrb.* 70 (1851): 110.

31. E. H. Ackerknecht, *Therapeutische Selbstversuche von Aerzten*, Documenta Geigy (Basle: Geigy, 1968).

32. L. M. Politzer, "Zur Kritik und Reform der Therapie," *Wien. Med. Wschr.* 26 (1876): 76ff.

The Appraisal of Analgesic Agents in Recent Decades: Prototype for the Study of Subjective Responses

Henry K. Beecher

General

We strive to go from individual experience to generality. We believe with Socrates that "genuine knowledge pertains only to universals." Bacon said the same thing in his phrase: "Philosophy discards individuals." Our overriding purpose in the past twenty years has been to seek out the general as it emerges from the particular. Thus our interest is broader than concern with the effect of analgesic agents on pain, broader even than the effect of central nervous system depressants in general on pain. We like to think of this as providing a workable prototype for the quantitative study of the effects of drugs on subjective responses in general.

As far as the central nervous system depressants go, we can see, for example, grounds for stating a unifying theory of action. Consider the sequence:

SEDATIVES – HYPNOTICS – ANALGESICS – EGO DEPRESSANTS – ANESTHETICS.

There are interrelationships of significance among these several effects of drugs. For example, the slightest mental depression produced by a barbiturate is sedation. Increase the dose of the same barbiturate and it becomes a hypnotic; sleep is produced. Increase the dose still further and the same barbiturate becomes a pain-relieving agent. Increase it still more and it is an ego depressant. A still further increase and it becomes an anesthetic agent. Thus by the simple expedient of increasing the dose of a given drug, in this case a barbiturate, one can pass from the slightest mental depression to the complete oblivion of anesthesia. It is impossible for me to believe that nature is aware of any of the interfaces between any of these categories. Therefore, what seems to me to be a sensible working assumption is that there must be mechanisms of action held in common by drugs that produce these states. One could then expect cross-fertilization of ideas from one drug to another. That is, we can learn about ego depressants by studying the sedatives, about anesthesia by studying analgesics, and so on. This has been the case.

There is a belief in some quarters, mostly theological, that science is cold and remote, concerned only with measurement. An opposite school, headed by Bentley Glass, holds that neither the processes nor the concepts of science are strictly objective. Certainly they are as objective as man knows how to make them. But science in the end is only man's way of looking at nature. As a human activity carried on by individual man or groups of men, it remains inescapably subjective. According to this school, science is ultimately as subjective as all other human knowledge, for it lives in the mind and the senses of the unique individual person. It is derived from man's subjective activities. "Mind is the mysterious substance which feels and thinks," according to John Stuart Mill, and, one could add, anticipates, wills, remembers—but Mill would doubtless say these are subsumed under "think." I am not interested in a semantic approach to these problems; I think it would be of very little profit to us in the present context. But I think that it is important to remind ourselves that all measurements are accomplished through the subjective characteristics of the individual. Nonetheless, we can speak of a quantitative approach to the elusive properties of the mind.

Psychopharmacology has its roots deeply buried in sensation and in alterations of sensations produced by drugs. It is thus inescapably subjective. The modern interest in scientific studies of sensation began 200 years ago with Haller's *Elementa Physiologiae* (1757–66), in which he discussed the senses fully. But it might be sounder to place the beginnings of the scientific interest in sensation at Charles Bell's discovery in 1811, and its confirmation 11 years later by Magendie, that there are two kinds of nerves: sensory, which lead to the posterior roots of the spinal cord, and motor, from the anterior roots. This discovery 150 years ago "reminded the physiologists that the mind's sensations were as much their business as the muscles' movements." Motor conduction could be studied 100 years ago, since the motor nerve has a muscle at its end. "At the end of a sensory nerve there was only introspection . . . ." (Boring, 1942.) However, present gaps in fundamental knowledge need not oblige us to remain at a purely descriptive level. We can now proceed from descriptive words alone to numbers, to quantification, in many instances in psychopharmacology, and I think it is urgent to do this whenever we can.

The beginnings of what Lord Kelvin might have called a scientific approach to these problems can be found in 1846. (You will recall that Lord Kelvin said: "I often say that when you can measure what you are speaking about and express it in numbers, you know something about it; but when you cannot measure it, when you cannot express it in numbers, your knowledge is of a meagre and unsatisfactory kind; it may be the beginning of knowledge, but you have scarcely, in your thoughts, advanced to the stage of *Science* whatever the matter may be.") In 1846 Ernst Heinrich Weber became interested in separating pain from the sensation of touch. Four years later, Fechner saw in Weber's studies on intensity of sensory experience a way of writing quantitative relations between mind and body, or, more particularly, between sensation and its stimulus (Boring, 1942). In all such studies of this kind one's bias may be crippling. The subjects' and the observers' bias must therefore be eliminated by the double blind approach. At times one must insert placebos, also as unknowns, with randomization of the placebos and drugs studied. I shall show a little later just how powerful these placebo effects can be. I shall also show you that *situations* can have placebo effects. One must enlarge the concept of a placebo from something that pleases to include the effects and situations produced by placebos which may be unpleasant. We must have isolation of one subject from another so that they cannot compare and discuss their experiences, lest the results be skewed. We must have mathematical validation of supposed differences, and a sufficient number of subjects, usually not fewer than twenty-five, for work on pain, for example.

"Experimental" Pain

When I set out twenty-six years ago to study pain and pain relief, I had no idea that one pain was different from another. Scores of studies had been made and scores of papers written on the subject. The war interrupted this work, and it was not until 1948 that Jane Denton and I started out on what we hoped would be an orderly study of the subject.

We started with the supposition that pain was pain, that it varied in duration, quality, and intensity, but that however it was produced it was pretty much the same thing, varying only in the qualities just mentioned. We knew that pain had been experimentally contrived in the laboratory in many ways: by skin pricks, by electric shocks to teeth, by chemicals placed in blisters, by tourniquets, by physical pressure, by cold, by heat. In the beginning we had no doubt that all of these methods were useful, for indeed they did produce pain—that was unquestionable. Thus we set out to use one of the methods which had been carefully worked out by Hardy, Wolff, and Goodell (1952). With our interest in quantification, this method was particularly attractive, for it presented a means of measuring accurately the amount of heat thrown on an area of the skin, usually the forehead. Since we wished to study pain in man, this seemed to be a fine approach. To cut short the story of a long and troublesome period, it was a rude shock for us to find that with this beautifully worked out method we could not distinguish between a large dose of morphine (15 mg.) and 1 ml. of normal saline when both of these agents were administered as unknowns to subject and observer. (This double-unknowns technique is a requirement in studies in this field.) We then turned to a man who had had a great deal of experience with this Hardy-Wolff-Goodell method and, again to shorten a long story, he was quite unable, notwithstanding his early successes with the method (when he had not worked with the double-unknowns technique), to distinguish between a large dose of morphine and a little table salt in solution.

As the years have gone by, some fifteen groups in Britain and the United States have utterly failed to demonstrate any dependable relationship in man between the relief of experimentally contrived pain and large doses of narcotic. This refers to the methods generally used at present. We supposed that it might be possible in the future to devise experimental methods wherein the pain threshold would respond in dependable fashion to graded doses of narcotic. These matters have all been dealt with extensively, with full references, in my book (Beecher, 1959). Our prediction has come true, as we shall see.

When this early failure of experimentally produced pain in man to respond dependably to even large doses of narcotic agents is taken into account, in conjunction with the universally observed fact that pain arising from disease or injury (what I shall call pathological pain) *always* responds in greater or lesser degree to even small doses of morphine and similar narcotics, it must be concluded that our original assumption that pain was pain whatever its origin simply does not hold. There is some fundamental and mysterious difference between pain (even severe pain) produced in the laboratory and the pain produced by disease or injury.

In fairness to Hardy, Wolff, and Goodell, and other originators of experimentally produced pain studies, I should like to say at once that experimentally contrived pain does have its uses in man. For example, the classic work of Gasser, Erlanger, Heinbecker, Bishop, and others, in which they identified pain pathways, has often depended upon experimentally produced pain. One must add also that experimental pain in animals is a useful approach to certain kinds of important studies. The Hardy-Wolff-Goodell method, for instance, works beautifully when a small quantity of heat is thrown on a rat's tail (D'Amour and Smith, 1941). I suspect that to an animal all pain is serious and significant, and that an animal is quite unable to distinguish between experimental pain and pathological pain. Indeed, there may be a clue in this statement to a significant factor in the pain situation. Later on, evidence will be given to indicate that the meaning of the pain sensation is the factor which determines the suffering from it. We all know that a small ache in a finger may be a trivial annoyance, easily disregarded, whereas the same duration and intensity of an ache beneath the sternum, if it connotes the possibility of sudden death from heart failure, may be a wholly unsettling experience. The implications contained in these statements are of such importance that I shall now deal with them in some detail.

Pathological Pain

It long ago became apparent from a study of the world's literature on pain that this subjective experience is one surrounded by many pitfalls to trap the unwary. It early became apparent that sound design of study was of paramount importance. Many workers have made contributions to this area.

For example, in Britain the Keeles (1948, 1952) long ago understood the requirements for study. Many important contributions have been made by colleagues in our laboratory, among them Denton, Lasagna, Keats, Gravenstein, and Smith. The contributions of many others, in addition to our own, have been described in my book (Beecher, 1959).

In our own work we chose to record whatever the fact was, severe pain for example, and to administer an unknown solution which might be either an active drug or a placebo; an unbiased technician visits the patient forty-five minutes and again ninety minutes after the drug is administered. For a positive result we arbitrarily require a patient to say his pain is at least half gone on both occasions. If he says it is all gone on one occasion and not half gone on another, this is arbitrarily recorded as a negative result.

There are many ways of approaching the problem; this one has worked well in our hands. It may seem that the "one-half gone" decision was a difficult one to make, but actual experience has shown that patients have found the judgment easy to make and to reproduce. We then take the number of individuals in a given group whose result was "positive" and calculate their percentage. This makes it possible to fulfil Lord Kelvin's requirement of placing significant numbers in front of meaningful items. We can thus compare a new agent with a standard—usually morphine—or a placebo in studies of pain.

That one can deal in a quantitative manner with this problem is demonstrated by data obtained in this laboratory (Keats, Beecher, and Mosteller, 1950). We had an outside individual make up two series of flasks, six flasks in series A and six in series B. We did not know what either series contained, but assumed that one series contained a pain-relieving agent. When we had completed the study, using postoperative wound pain, and broke the code, we found that both series of flasks had contained morphine. In series A there was always 10 mg. per ml. In series B there were different concentrations of morphine in each flask. On graphing the data we constructed the two lines shown in Figure 1. Where the two graphs cross, there is equivalence of analgesic action: we had equated 10 mg. of morphine to 10.8—a 9 per cent error. As any statistician knows, these are not truly lines that cross, but bands that cross, and the regression lines have to be calculated. This was done under the guidance

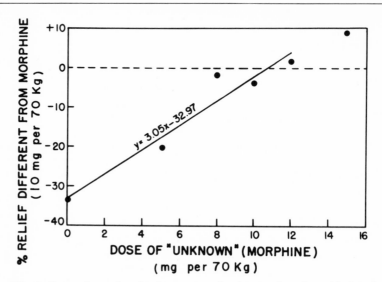

Fig. 1. Comparison of analgesic potency of unknown drug (morphine) and of morphine (Keats, Beecher, and Mosteller, 1950).

of Professor Frederick Mosteller, without whom none of our work would have been possible. These calculations required that we add 2 per cent more to the 9 per cent error and give a total error of 11 per cent. We are thus able to work quantitatively in the elusive field of subjective responses. I submit that this 11 per cent error is about as accurate a measurement as one can obtain with most of the objective things in man (except, perhaps, for chemical determinations in a sample of blood) such as blood pressure or cell counts.

The Marshall-Strong Concept

In 1894, the philosopher Marshall wrote a book, *Pain, Pleasure and Aesthetics*, in which he almost made a crucial assumption. He did in fact lay the ground for an assumption that was made the next year by Strong (1895). This assumption, in effect, was that an experience such as suffering has two major components: the original sensation and the processing component, or what I like to call the psychological reaction component. So far as I have been able to discover, neither Marshall nor Strong had any factual evidence for this concept. It seems to have been simply one of those brilliant intuitive insights which have been so rewarding in medicine over the centuries. We have been able to gain, however, considerable supporting evidence for this Marshall-Strong concept—evidence that has given us some rather far-reaching insights not only into the origins of pain and the control of pain but also into other subjective responses and their modification by drugs in man.

The Reaction Component

I have already mentioned that an experience such as suffering consists of two elements, the original sensation and the reaction component, and that pain as now commonly contrived experimentally does not respond in man in a dependable fashion to even large doses of narcotics. From this evolved the working hypothesis that the original sensation was not the site of action of drugs such as morphine. It is surely true that there is no such thing as pure sensation, all sensations having been modified, probably at a subcortical level before they erupt into consciousness and certainly after erupting into consciousness, by conditioning, significance, and meaning. If, as seems to be the case, agents such as narcotics are without effect on the original sensation, then the site of action must be the reaction component. At least we can take this as a working hypothesis and then see how pertinent data relate to the concept. I now propose to present evidence that the reaction component has a vast influence on our lives.

Placebos

It was only after I had worked in this field for some years that I realized that we usually had a high average degree of effectiveness of placebos in treating postoperative wound pain, and other conditions as well. Following this realization, I looked around among the reports of other individuals and was struck by the beautiful study of Evans and Hoyle (1933) in England. In this pioneer and now classic study they found that the pain of angina pectoris was relieved by placebos just about as often as we later found for the pain of postoperative wounds. This article of Evans and Hoyle marks a considerable milestone in clinical sophistication in studies of subjective responses. The results of a further search for other comparable findings have been summarized elsewhere (Beecher, 1959).

On the average, the relief produced by placebos in pathological pain is indistinguishable from that produced by an "active" drug in about 35 per cent of cases, whereas the average effectiveness of placebos with experimentally contrived pain is only 3.2 per cent. In other words, the placebo is *ten times* more effective in relieving pain of pathological origin than it is in relieving pain of experimentally contrived origin. There is some evidence, moreover, that, when stress is severe, the effectiveness of placebos increases greatly, and may even double. These data, I believe, are difficult to ignore, and they illustrate my point. There is, it is true, an assumption here, but one I do not believe anybody would have difficulty in accepting, that there is more anxiety associated with pain from disease than there is in pain experimentally contrived in the laboratory. This assumption seems to be so far removed from the possibility of adequate challenge that it need not be discussed further. In other words, when stress is severe, placebos are more effective than when stress is mild or absent.

I mentioned earlier that morphine was not dependably effective in man in relieving experimentally contrived pain as usually produced, but was always effective in greater or lesser degree in relieving pain of pathological origin. Thus one can, I believe, state a new principle of drug action: some drugs are effective only in the presence of an appropriate mental state.

Much more could be said about chemical agents as placebos, but before we leave this section, I should like to point out that situations can also have placebo effects: the surgical situation, for example. In 1939 it was suggested, in Italy, that the pain of angina pectoris could be greatly lessened by ligation of the internal mammary arteries. Eventually this suggestion was adopted in the United States and quite spectacularly favorable results were obtained. Not only were the objective results impressive, but the patients said they felt better, and the objective evidence supported this: there was great reduction in the number of nitroglycerin tablets taken, and exercise tolerance was greatly increased. One patient, for example, could take only four minutes of standardized exercise before intolerable pain stopped him and the T-waves in his electrocardiogram inverted in an ominous way. After the operation he could exercise for ten minutes without pain on the exercise steps and his T-waves did not invert.

Several individuals (compare Cobb et al., 1959; Dimond et al., 1958; Adams, 1958; and Fish et al., 1958) began to wonder if this might not be a placebo effect. They therefore went to their patients, explained the situation, and told them they would like to carry out a study in which the patients would not know what had been done, nor would the observers know until the study was completed. They told their patients that half of them would have the internal mammary arteries exposed and ligated and the other half would simply have them exposed but not ligated. These studies were carried out, and, in the case I have just mentioned, the patient with intolerable pain after four minutes of exercise, who after the operation could stand ten minutes of exercise, had had only the sham operation. Many similar examples indicated that ligation had no real effect beyond that of a placebo. The difficulty in the present situation was that, even though the operation was innocuous in concept, individuals with angina pectoris are in a vulnerable state: one patient died during the procedure and another had a further severe myocardial infarction. Even this simple procedure was not without real hazard. This hazard might have been tolerable if the placebo effects had been lasting, but unfortunately, placebo effects usually last only from days to weeks, or to months at best. Thus we have an example of a situation rather than a chemical agent acting as a placebo. We should all make a searching examination of our present procedures to see which surgical operations or medical activities at the present time may possibly be nothing more than placebo procedures (Beecher, 1961, 1962). Placebo effects, however produced, are surely to be construed as evidence for the existence of a powerful reaction component.

A New Class of Analgesic Agents

I am sure I do not need to point out the anecdotal nature of my remarks. My excuse, if I need one, is that I was directed to delve into personal history, and history is often anecdotal. In this vein I should like to mention an observation made by Lasagna and myself in 1954 that surprised us as much as anyone else. Actually, two things surprised us, that most workers using nalorphine had failed to produce any effect in animals but that it was powerfully effective as an analgesic in man. Unfortunately this agent had such severe hallucinogenic effects that it was useless clinically as an analgesic. It had another value, however: our finding directed the study of analgesics into a new and unanticipated but promising direction toward the morphine antagonists. The search goes on for agents in this class that will be nonaddicting, without the severe side effects we encountered, but yet powerful as an analgesic.

At Last A Useful Experimental Pain Method

To the best of my knowledge no one had heretofore presented acceptable dose-effect curves for narcotics and experimentally contrived pain in man. It is perhaps not necessary to review the well-known failures, including our own, to put the tourniquet method on a sound basis. The method has had a long and unsatisfactory history. However, Smith, Egbert, Markowitz, Mosteller, and myself have now modified the method so that it dependably differentiates morphine from a placebo. This method involves a limited period of exercise with the tourniquet in place and the buildup of pain with the passage of time. The time required to achieve slight, moderately distressing, very distressing, and unbearable pain is recorded. Intravenous morphine, 10 mg. per 70 kg. of body weight, was found to delay significantly the top three grades of pain in man (Fig. 2), but all three were at the same percentage level. The magnitude of the morphine effect was approximately a fixed multiple of the score $(M - P)/P$; this equals approximately 0.7 in all pain categories except "slight." One hesitates, therefore, to conclude that there are important *qualitative*

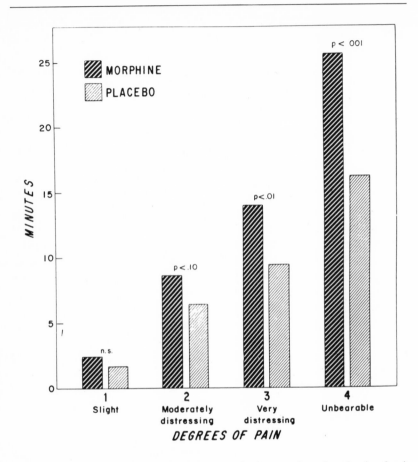

Fig. 2. Mean duration of stimulation required to produce four levels of pain after morphine (10 mg. per 70 kg. body weight) and after placebo. (Derived from unpublished material by G. M. Smith and co-workers.

differences between slight and severe pain beyond the fact that the data for slight pain have the quality of considerable variability, while the data for severe pain have the quality of comparative stability. Nonetheless, common sense indicates that there is greater stress (anxiety) present in the severe pain group than there is with slight pain.

Tourniquet pain more closely resembles pathological pain than pain produced by other experimental pain methods. It builds up slowly and persists, whereas most experimental pain methods involve only quick stabs or jabs of pain. These, of course, somewhat resemble the colics or angina, notoriously difficult for some unclear reason to allay with even powerful narcotics. Smith and associates believe that tourniquet pain can be made to resemble pathological pain, even more closely than has yet been done, by not allowing the subject to terminate the pain, just as pathological pain cannot be terminated at will. This, of course, will require a hardy group of subjects who will agree to such participation.

There are several kinds of dose-effect curves. Two important ones are studies of the effect of a given dose of narcotic on several degrees of pain (Fig. 2), as used by Smith and associates; and what might be called the classic dose-effect curve obtained by studying the response of a steady degree of pain to different doses of narcotic. Work on this is under way at present. I do not believe that one type of dose-effect curve could be true and the other false. Some caution is necessary, however. Perhaps it is not really necessary to determine both types, but at this stage it seems better to obtain both.

It can be seen in Figure 2 that significant differences emerge only when the upper grades of pain are reached. Perhaps we can see in this why experimental pain methods in man have been so undependable; they have almost universally dealt with slight pain, with threshold pain. The root of the problem here probably is the great variability of these data at the low level.

In conclusion, one can speculate about what is at the bottom of the difference between the two pain levels, slight and severe. It is,'I believe, anxiety. Several things that I have mentioned fit in with this view.

1. Experimental pain methods were easily shown to be useful in animals. To an animal all pain is undoubtedly serious and meaningful.

2. Wikler and his associates, using experimental pain, found a dependable difference between narcotic and placebo when anxiety was interjected into the situation.

3. My wartime observations on the Anzio beachhead seem pertinent. Despite severe wounds, the soldiers experienced less suffering (the wound meant escape from an intolerable situation and was seemingly construed as a good thing) than did civilians who experienced the disaster of requiring surgery.

4. There is a ten-fold greater effectiveness of placebos when pathological pain is dealt with than there is with experimental pain. One assumes, reasonably enough I think, that pain of pathological origin is associated with more anxiety than is experimentally contrived pain in man.

Conclusion

Measurement in the field of sensations and mood presents an area of significance in human behavior. This work is a relevant bridge between psychopharmacology and the behavioral sciences. The behavioral sciences must, if they are to be soundly established, move onward from the present state, which in many areas is largely one of description, to one of measurement. Measurement depends upon the recognition and precise definition of variables and their relationships, and the development of tools and techniques for working with them in quantitative terms. As in all sciences, eventually there must be possibilities of prediction. Implicit in this is the necessity not only to recognize elements that can be measured but to understand the existence and nature of the essential safeguards, the controls, of observations made. One goal of science is rules ("laws"), and the more invariable these rules are, the better it is. We seek to predict from given situation to certain effect. In the complex field of the behavioral sciences in man, observations have, as mentioned, so far been largely descriptive. The basic purpose of these remarks is to show that a quantitative approach to sensation ("feeling") is possible and rewarding. Sensation as used here, and mood, are often controlling factors in behavior and as such are elementary considerations in the development of the behavioral sciences.

References

Adams, R. 1958. Internal-mammary-artery ligation for coronary insufficiency. *New Eng. J. Med.* 258: 113–15.
Beecher, H. K. 1959. Measurement of subjective responses: Quantitative effects of drugs. New York: Oxford University Press.
Beecher, H. K. 1961. Surgery as placebo. A quantitative study of bias. *J.A.M.A.* 176: 1102–7.
Beecher, H. K. 1962. Nonspecific forces surrounding disease and the treatment of disease. *J.A.M.A.* 179: 437–40.
Boring, E. G. 1942. Sensation and perception in the history of experimental psychology. New York: Appleton-Century-Crofts.
Cobb, L. A., Thomas, G. I., Dillard, D. H., Merendino, K. A., and Bruce, R. A. 1959. An evaluation of internal-mammary-artery ligation by a double-blind technic. *New Eng. J. Med.* 260: 1115–18.
D'Amour, F. E., and Smith, D. L. 1941. A method for determining loss of pain sensation. *J. Pharmacol.* 72: 74–79.
Dimond, E. G., Kittle, C. F., and Crockett, J. E. 1958. Evaluation of internal artery ligation and sham procedure in angina pectoris. *Circulation* 18: 712–13.
Evans, W., and Hoyle, C. 1933. The comparative value of drugs used in the continuous treatment of angina pectoris. *Quart. J. Med.* 2: 311–38.
Fish, R. G., Crymes, T. P., and Lovell, M. G. 1958. Internal-mammary-artery ligation for angina pectoris. Its failure to produce relief. *New Eng. J. Med.* 259: 418–20.
Hardy, J. D., Wolff, H. G., and Goodell, H. 1952. Pain sensations and reactions. Baltimore: Williams & Wilkins Co.
Hill, H. E., Kornetsky, C. H., Flanary, H. G., and Wikler, A. 1952. Effects of anxiety and morphine on discrimination of intensities of painful stimuli. *J. Clin. Invest.* 31: 473–80.
Hill, H. E., Kornetsky, C. H., Flanary, H. G., and Wikler, A. 1952. Studies on anxiety associated with anticipation of pain. I. Effects of morphine. *Arch. Neurol. Psychiat.* 67: 612–19.

Keats, A. S., Beecher, H. K., and Mosteller, F. C. 1950. Measurement of pathological pain in distinction to experimental pain. *J. Appl. Physiol.* 3: 35–44.

Keele, C. A. 1952. The assay of analgesic drugs on man. *Analyst* 77: 111–17.

Keele, K. D. 1948. The pain chart. *Lancet* 2: 6–8.

Kornetsky, C. 1954. Effects of anxiety and morphine on the anticipation and perception of painful radiant thermal stimuli. *J. Comp. Physiol. Psychol.* 47: 130–32.

Lasagna, L., and Beecher, H. K. 1954. The analgesic effectiveness of nalorphine and nalorphine-morphine combinations in man. *J. Pharmacol. Exp. Ther.* 112: 356–63.

Marshall, H. R. 1894. Pain, pleasure, and aesthetics. London: Macmillan.

Smith, G. M., Egbert, L. D., Markowitz, R. A., Mosteller, F., and Beecher, H. K. 1966. An experimental pain method sensitive to morphine in man: the submaximum effort tourniquet technique. *J. Pharmacol. Exp. Ther.* 154: 324–32.

Smith, G. M., Lowenstein, E., and Beecher, H. K. Unpublished data.

Strong, C. A. 1895. The psychology of pain. *Psychol. Rev.* 2: 329–47.

The Role of the
Pharmaceutical Industry

David L. Cowen

The role of the pharmaceutical industry in the control of drugs—and I interpret control liberally as involving the determination of what drugs are made available, the determination of the over-all quality of those drugs, and the determination of the forms in which the drugs are dispensed—was inherent in the circumstances of the nineteenth-century origins of the industry and the social forces at work during its formative years. Those origins were in the pharmacy shop and the chemical plant; the molding forces were the burgeoning industrial revolution and the tremendous scientific explosion.

The early industry, in France, the United States, Germany, and England, and undoubtedly elsewhere, took over from the pharmacy shop the task of making galenicals, especially in the form of fluidextracts. This last was a dosage form which the pharmacist could readily concoct individually. The industry was forced, therefore, to assume the responsibility of providing drugs of a kind, quality, and efficacy sufficient to persuade the pharmacist, despite his understandable opposition, to give up his birthright. This was a responsibility that set the tenor of the industry's role thereafter.

A few illustrations will make this clear.* In Germany, Eugen Dieterich, the founder of the Fabrik Helfenberg, talking of his experience with his plant for the manufacture of galenicals (founded in 1869), pointed out that success had come only after he had built appropriate machinery, devised appropriate manufacturing processes, and found effective scientific means of critically evaluating not only the finished product but also the raw materials. "Manufacturing on a scientific basis," Dieterich said, "would develop the ideal side of my activity, perfected through a highly developed pharmaceutical technique." [1] Dieterich was certainly a pioneer in the scientific control of galenicals, and success came from his efficient production of scientifically superior products. [2]

* This paper cannot pretend to be a comprehensive history of the industry. The illustrations are just that, and no claim of priority or exclusiveness can necessarily be attributed to them.

1. Quoted by W. Schneider, "Aus der Geschichte der deutschen pharmazeutischen Industrie im 19. Jahrhundert," reprint from 23rd International Congress of Pharmaceutical Sciences, Münster/Westfalen, 1963, *Tagungsheft*, p. 3.

2. Communication to the author from Dr. Georg Dann, Kiel.

In the United States, also in 1869, Parke, Davis & Company had begun the manufacture of fluidextracts. In 1879 the company had boasted that it had standardized its "Liquor Ergotae Purificatus" by the precipitation of the organic acid with lead acetate. This was certainly a very early, if not the earliest, attempt at providing uniformity in this kind of product, and it was followed by a series of products dubbed "normal liquids," whose uniformity was assured by the use of Mayer's reagent.[3] Regardless of the effectiveness and actual accomplishment of these procedures, here was an approach to drug control by which the industry placed itself beyond the reach of the individual practitioner of medicine or pharmacy. The success attained by the industry is amply demonstrated by the catalogue of G. D. Searle which was offering, late in the 1880's, 400 fluidextracts, 150 elixirs, 100 syrups, 75 powdered extracts, 25 tinctures, and other drug forms for which claims of uniformity of potency and action were made.[4]

Parke, Davis & Company went one step further: the practitioner might or might not be influenced by claims of uniformity, elegance, and economy, but he could not very long disregard new remedies of purported efficacy. In 1874 agents were first sent afield to search out crude drugs. From the West Coast, from many parts of North and South America, from Fiji and elsewhere, came crude drugs from which fluidextracts were made and "distributed to physicians."[5] By 1880, forty-eight such new products were available, some of which remained in the pharmacopoeia for a long time. Although no clinical tests on animals or humans were involved—physicians were urged to report their results to the company—the industry had been taught the commercial, if not the medical, effectiveness of providing new drugs.

From the pharmacy shop stemmed another and quite different aspect of the pharmaceutical industry. The work of a large number of pharmacists in Sweden, Germany, and France with the vegetable alkaloids and the halogens late in the eighteenth century and early in the nineteenth opened up new paths for industrialization. We need not recount the therapeutic revolution, if not explosion, that followed the introduction of morphine and quinine, iodoform, chloral hydrate, and ethylchloride. The innumerable vegetable alkaloids provided a rationale for the old herbalism; the halogen derivatives, a modern approach to chemiatrics. More to our interest here is that this revolution brought with it industrialization, and that while the pharmacist continued to

3. F. O. Taylor, "Forty-five Years of Manufacturing Pharmacy," *J. Amer. Pharm. Ass.* 4 (1915): 471, 473; "They Made Drug Therapy Reliable," *Ther. Notes* (June, 1941), pp. 184–89.

4. M. L. Tainter and G. M. A. Marcelli, "Rise of Synthetic Drugs in the American Pharmaceutical Industry," *Bull. N.Y. Acad. Med.* 35 (1959): 396.

5. Taylor, "Forty-five Years," pp. 470, 471.

isolate active principles and to develop halogen compounds, it was the industry that took over the role of producer.

Here again we have the rudimentary beginnings of one of industry's roles—the production and development of the fruits of the labors of private investigators. But there is more, for while the pharmacist could adopt the industrial product or continue to compound his own galenicals according to his own convenience, he had virtually no choice with the alkaloids. The alkaloids were highly powerful and often poisonous substances that could not be isolated by everyday techniques and equipment. Purity was especially important, and, although the alkaloids could readily be purified, the cost made it unprofitable for the individual operator to undertake the task.[6] Moreover, the alkaloids were provided in a form that made possible a quantification in dosage not obtainable before. Industrialization thus was almost inevitable, and the industry gave evidence of its potential to produce pharmaceuticals of good quality economically and—perhaps of particular significance here—in quantities large enough to meet the health needs of society.

Thus far we have discussed the role of the industry as it derived from, and, in large measure, began to assume the functions of, the pharmacy shop. The industry, as noted at the outset, grew out of the chemical plant as well as out of the pharmacy, especially after chemistry itself had progressed to the stage of working with cyclical compounds. Carbolic acid, salicylic acid, phenacetin, and the antipyretics were synthetic chemicals which the laboratory in the back of the pharmacy shop could produce even less satisfactorily than it could the organic alkaloidal chemicals. The turn the German synthetic chemical industry took toward the production of pharmaceuticals had its starting point in Kolbe's successful development of a relatively economic process for the production of salicylic acid in 1874 (the chemical itself had been known since 1837).[7] Here was an entirely new role for pharmaceutical research, in and out of the industry—the creation of substances of therapeutic value that did not occur in nature. Here began the molecular manipulation, or "improvement" as the industry publicists prefer to call it, which sought to create new, or more efficacious, or less toxic, agents. This type of chemical procedure was adaptable to the organic chemicals as well, as shown by Ladenburg's development of homatropine out of atropine in 1880 and Knoll's development of codeine from morphine in 1886.[8]

But the introduction of new chemical entities into therapeutics, whether they came from original organic sources or were synthetic,

6. See Schneider, "Aus der Geschichte," p. 8.
7. *The Dispensatory of the United States*, 15th ed., H. C. Wood, *et al.*, eds. (Philadelphia: J. B. Lippincott, 1883), p. 98.
8. Schneider, "Aus der Geschichte," p. 8.

again forced industry to assume an additional responsibility. Whereas three years after the introduction of homatropine it could still be said that the action of this drug upon the system had not been studied,[9] the introduction of entities for which there was no so-called empirical or traditional basis cried out for some sort of proof of safety and efficacy before, and control during, the test of the substance in the human body. The process was not entirely voluntary; deaths during the early use of diphtheria antitoxin caused health officials to insist upon some form of testing and control of sera.[10]

The new science of pharmacology came to the rescue and provided the industry with a working basis for preliminary testing. It is difficult to say when pharmacology stepped out of the laboratories of the institutes and universities, that is, when exactly the ideas and techniques of Magendie and Bernard, and especially of Oswald Schmiederberg, perhaps the first to subject the traditions of the materia medica to pharmacological tests in 1872,[11] began to infiltrate the industrial laboratory. In 1894 or later, Parke, Davis & Company, following the trend toward increased attention to pharmacology in medical education, established a small department of pharmacology. Originally intended for the production of diphtheria antitoxin, the laboratory was put into the charge of two bacteriologists from the University of Michigan. Guinea pigs, cocks, and dogs were used, and E. M. Houghton, claiming to follow Ehrlich's lead, introduced the frog-heart test to assay drugs such as digitalis and strophanthus.[12] If, however, we are to judge from the facts that Hoechst in Germany seems to have had no pharmacological facilities to help Ehrlich and Von Behring in their efforts to standardize diphtheria antitoxin,[13] and that Eli Lilly had no pharmacological laboratory until 1929, nor Merck and Company until 1933,[14] it must be concluded that pharmacological testing remained until relatively recently a function of more or less private laboratories.

A second method of testing drugs is, of course, the clinical test. Here again the time of its becoming an obligation of the industry is difficult

9. *Dispensatory of the United States*, p. 284n.
10. W. Greiling, *Im Banne der Medizin: Paul Ehrlich, Leben und Werk* (Düsseldorf: Econ-Verlag, 1954), p. 35.
11. C. A. Keele, "Empiricism and Logic in the Discovery of New Drugs," *Nature* (London) 195 (1962): 639; C. F. Schmidt, "The Old and the New in Therapeutics," *Circ. Res.* 8 (1960): 687.
12. Taylor, "Forty-five Years," p. 479; "They Made Drug Therapy Reliable," pp. 184–89.
13. Koch gave a goat and a lamb to Ehrlich and Von Behring; they were obliged to purchase other animals out of their own resources. Greiling, *Im Banne der Medizin*, p. 26.
14. V. A. Drill, "Basic Research in the Pharmaceutical Industry," *J. Indiana Med. Ass.* 55 (1962): 69.

to ascertain. Parke, Davis' distribution of new extracts to physicians and the publication of their reports as they became available, in the 1880's, can hardly qualify as clinical testing.[15] Hoechst's work with the antipyretics began after Wilhelm Filehne had, in 1882, put the first synthetic of this class, kairine, through a series of clinical tests with healthy persons and had experimented with dosages on sick patients.[16] Similar activity was thereafter common, to judge by Von Behring's work with diphtheria antitoxin, and later Ehrlich's work with salvarsan. (In passing, the chemist–pharmacologist–industrial-producer sequence with regard to kairine is worth noting. Kairine had been synthesized by Otto Fischer at the Hochschule in Munich, its medicinal potential had been recognized by Filehne, then Professor of Materia Medica at Erlangen, and it was eventually put into production by Hoechst.[17])

There remains to be described one other role that the pharmaceutical industry had undertaken in the nineteenth century—its development of new dosage forms. Again the industry learned from the pharmacist, and again the end results were forms which the individual pharmacist could duplicate, if at all, only at the cost of considerable labor.

For example, pills were sugar coated in France in the 1830's and produced successfully on a large scale in the United States by William Warner in 1866;[18] "pearl-coated" pills were manufactured by the developer Arthur Cox in England in the 1840's.[19] Compressed tablets, perhaps the one dosage form whose development depended primarily on technological innovations such as simple hand-punches and automatic power machines, also were introduced.[20] Gelatin capsules, which had their origins in France where the pharmacist A. Mothes made a crude prototype, and which soon thereafter came into use in the United States, did not become significant until Parke, Davis & Company undertook to have them manufactured on a large scale about 1875.[21]

Warner also introduced the "parvule" into American practice in 1879. The firm of Abbott Laboratories in 1891 introduced the "dosimetric granule," a dosage form derived from the work of Adolph Burggraeve in Paris, which French manufacturers were already seeking to market in the

15. G. S. Bender, "The Making of Better Medicines" (Unpublished MS., Parke, Davis & Co.), pp. 4–5.

16. W. Filehne, "Über neue Mittel, welche die fieberhafte Temperatur zur Norm bringen" (1882–83), reprinted in *Wie die ersten Heilmittel nach Hoechst kamen*, Dokumente aus Hoechster Archiven, no. 8 (Frankfurt/M: Hoechst, 1965), p. 15; and the introduction to these *Dokumente*, p. 8.

17. *Ibid.*, pp. 7, 8, 10, 13.

18. G. Sonnedecker, *Kremens and Urdang's History of Pharmacy*, 3d ed. (Philadelphia: Lippincott, 1963), p. 288.

19. *Chemist and Druggist Centenary Number* (Nov. 10, 1959), p. 194.

20. Sonnedecker, *History of Pharmacy*, p. 289.

21. Taylor, "Forty-five Years," pp. 477–78.

United States. The dosimetric granule presented another idea which could better be carried out by industrial practices than by the individual worker, namely, that the medication should consist of chemically pure, stable, and precisely manufactured dosages, uniform in quality and quantity.[22]

Still another dosage form was the ampoule. Also the invention of a French pharmacist, Stanislas Limousin, this device enabled the industry to provide the physician with so great a variety of injectable solutions that it is hardly surprising that for a while he became hypodermic-needle-happy.[23]

Finally, note must be made of the development of biologicals. Completely beyond the pharmacist or physician, the production of sera, toxins, and antitoxins taxed even the capacity of industry, and industry again was in a position to increase its power over the substance of the materia medica. For example, Hoechst immediately took over the manufacture of Von Behring's diphtheria antitoxin.[24]

In the last decade of the nineteenth century and the first third of the twentieth, two new developments took place that enhanced the role of the pharmaceutical industry. One was the introduction of research laboratories, the other the introduction of quality control techniques. Together these two were to make almost unassailable either in quantity or in quality the industry's control over the production of drugs.

The beginnings of the research, or more correctly the research and development, laboratories of the pharmaceutical industry are obscure. They seem to have originated in Germany, at least the laboratories devoted to chemical synthesis. Hoechst, however, does not date its "scientific tradition" until the arrival of Ludwig Knorr in 1883.[25] It was World War I that stimulated industrial (and academic) drug research in Britain.[26] In the United States, Parke, Davis boasts of having had a research building as early as 1902, and Abbott places its first concerted research activity at about 1925, but Max Tishler has properly placed the "introduction of *modern* research" into the industry in the decade of the 1930's.[27]

The research in these laboratories, which bring together chemists,

22. H. Kogan, *The Long White Line* (New York: Random House, 1963), pp. 11–15.
23. See D. L. Cowen, *Medicine and Health in New Jersey: A History* (Princeton: D. Van Nostrand, 1964), pp. 49–50.
24. H. Satter, *Paul Ehrlich* (Munich, 1962), p. 52.
25. *Ludwig Knorr Begründer Hoechster wissenschaftlicher Tradition*, Dokumente aus Hoechster Archiven, no. 31 (Frankfurt/M: Hoechst, 1968), p. 7.
26. A. Duckworth, "Rise of the Pharmaceutical Industry," *Chemist and Druggist Centenary Number* (Nov. 10, 1959), p. 130.
27. F. O. Taylor, "Parke, Davis and Company," *Industr. Engineer. Chem.* 19 (1927): 1209; Kogan, *Long White Line*, pp. 112, 120; M. Tishler, "Role of the Drug House in Biological and Medical Research," *Bull. N.Y. Acad. Med.* 35 (1959): 593.

biochemists, microbiologists, pharmacologists, pathologists, physicians, and other specialists, has become the mainstay of the large pharmaceutical house. It is estimated that in 1968 American industrial expenditures for research reached $500,000,000.[28] This research is directed essentially toward the creation of new products; it is applied research, which is, however, to an appreciable extent nourished by basic research.[29]

From these research laboratories come new entities, new combinations of drugs, new dosage forms, and, perhaps most important, chemical syntheses of new entities. The nineteenth century saw the industry gaining control of drug production because of its success, real or reputed, in developing uniform, pure, and efficacious products. The twentieth, reflecting both improvements in science and technology and the imposition of governmental restraints, saw these therapeutic requirements augmented by, and more precisely defined in terms of, standards for drug characteristics such as potency, speed of action, rate of absorption, and rate of elimination.[30] The quest for understanding the mechanisms of drugs not only added a new dimension to therapeutics but opened the way for a "rational pharmacology," potentially capable of developing made-to-measure medicinal agents.[31] Attached to or associated with such research laboratories are arrangements, supported by the industry, for the clinical testing of new developments. This segment of research is concerned essentially with problems of efficacy, therapeutic ratio, and toxicity.

Science as a handmaiden of industry has also been made to serve, along with technology, in the quality control of products of the industry. Rudiments of quality control procedures were introduced into the pharmaceutical industry late in the nineteenth century. Johnson & Johnson, for example, created "scientific laboratories" in 1889 that included among their manifold functions the inspection of finished products.[32] This sort of inspection constituted what the quality control engineer calls the "first formal approach to quality control," but not until the 1920's did modern scientific quality control begin to make headway, and not until the 1950's did the concept of "total quality control" take hold.[33] Complex

28. American Medical Association, *Report of the Commission on Research* (Chicago: A.M.A., 1967), p. 30.
29. On basic research done by industry, see C. A. Keele, "Empiricism and Logic in the Discovery of New Drugs," *Nature* (London) 195 (1962): 642; J. C. Fischer, "Basic Research in Industry," *Science* 129 (1959): 1653–57. However, it must be noted that criticisms that industry does not do sufficient basic research are frequently heard.
30. See W. Modell, "The Basis for the Choice and Use of New Drugs," *GP* 20 (1959): 13.
31. See D. W. Woolley, "The Revolution in Pharmacology," *Perspect. Biol. Med.* 1 (1958): 174–97.
32. D. L. Cowen, "Two Outstanding New Jersey Pharmacists," *New Jersey J. Pharm.* 37 (Oct., 1964): 27.
33. R. A. Freund, "Quality Control—A Decade of Progress," *Industr. Qual. Contr.* 22 (1965): 67–68.

manufacturing processes in the pharmaceutical industry, and the special medicinal character of the products, made exacting quality testing procedures imperative. These were concerned not only with ascertaining the therapeutic integrity of the final product but also with such characteristics as particle size, stability, dissolution rate, hydrating or dehydrating capacities, and viscosity. Special procedures provided for control of raw materials, biologicals, and microbiologicals as well.[34]

Despite the fact that neither industrial research nor quality control advanced very far in the first third of the century, the industry had some considerable success with sera and antitoxins, with the chemotherapeutic agent salvarsan, and with hormones and vitamins. More important, the development of research and control apparatus prepared the way, or had to be developed in order to be ready, for the therapeutic explosion that followed the introduction of the sulfa group of chemotherapeutic agents and of the antibiotics in the 1930's and 1940's. The steady stream of magic bullets and miracle drugs that our generation has seen is truly remarkable. One can only come out with a sense of accomplishment in contemplating the various classes of drugs that attack infection and correct or palliate a great variety of organic and systemic malfunctions.

This discussion has so far seemed to place in the hands of the industry the control of drugs, as defined at the outset, without considering the existence of other, admittedly potent, loci of control. Certainly, the government, the medical profession, and private and university research agencies are not without influence in the determination of what drugs are made available. Certainly governments have made and are making requirements of safety and efficacy, and certainly there is ongoing nonindustrial research of even larger proportions than that in industry. Nevertheless, the relative freedom of choice enjoyed by the industry as to what it will and will not research, develop, or produce largely determines what the practitioner's armamentarium shall consist of. This may often prove of inestimable value to therapeutics. Smith Kline & French spent many years hunting for an antihistamine and eventually, even if somewhat fortuitously, helped to open up the whole field of tranquilizers; Merck Sharp & Dohme embarked on a time-consuming program of basic research on the kidney and opened up a whole field of diuretics. This freedom, it must be noted, does not always have a salutary effect. The proliferation of drugs that offer no new therapeutic advantage and the high-powered merchandising of drugs that seek to take advantage of economic opportunity rather than to meet a medical need may serve only

34. The ramifications of present-day quality control are detailed in W. S. Felker, "Quality Control in the Pharmaceutical Industry," *Drug Cosmet. Industr.* 91 (1962): 702ff, *passim*, and in the discussion of this paper, which Felker presented to an F.I.P. symposium, in *Pharm. Industr.* 25 (1963): 59–61. I am indebted to Dr. Herbert Wietschoreck of Hoechst for calling these to my attention.

to confuse the physician and to increase unnecessarily the use and the cost of drugs.

It is of even greater significance that the industry may determine what does *not* get into the physician's armamentarium. Evidence indicates that the production of penicillin and polio vaccine,[35] and the participation of industry in cancer research[36] and in mental health research,[37] were all circumscribed by industry's desire to protect its own economic interests. There is always the fear, according to one of the more enlightened industrial leaders, that governmental patent policies may "rob all pharmaceutical firms participating in the N.I.H. program of the necessary incentives to develop, produce, and market the product which might emerge."[38] I do not intend to indict the industry on this score; I intend only to point up the control that industry can exert in a profit economy on the availability or lack of availability of drugs.

Industry has arrogated to itself a considerable amount of the credit for the therapeutic revolution that has taken place. Some of this is deserved, but much of it is the result of promotional exaggerations and sophistries that do violence to one's sense of history. To take an extreme example, there is the recent statement of an industrial spokesman to the effect that in seeking "some examples of drugs originated by firms, I quickly found that practically none came from anywhere else."[39] I might direct this gentleman to William Withering and Edward Jenner, to John Abel and Edward Kendall, to Jonas Salk and A. B. Sabin. I might remind him that Merck of Darmstadt had a host of original contributions of pharmacists like Sertürner to work with; that Hoechst had its Fischer and Filehne for its antipyretics, Von Behring for diphtheria antitoxin, and Ehrlich for salvarsan; that Eli Lilly had Banting and Best for insulin; that Merck Sharp & Dohme had Hench for corticosteroids, and Waksman for streptomycin; that Abbott had Roger Adams for Veronal and Novocain; and that Parke, Davis had Burkholder for Chloromycetin. E. B. Chain[40] and Max Tishler,[41] both highly complimentary to industry for the role it has played,

35. U.S. District Court for the District of New Jersey. Criminal Action No. 173–58. *U.S.A.* v. *Eli Lilly & Co.*, *et al.* Trial Brief for the United States (mimeographed), p. 4.

36. Paul Talalay, *Drugs in Our Society* (Baltimore: Johns Hopkins Press, 1964), p. 289.

37. U.S. Congress, Senate, Committee on the Judiciary, *Administered Prices; Hearings before the Subcommittee on Antitrust and Monopoly* (Estes Kefauver, Chairman), 86th Cong., 2d sess., Jan. 21–29, 1960, pt. 16, "Administered Prices in the Drug Industry" (Washington: Government Printing Office, 1960), pp. 8995–96.

38. J. T. Connor, "Government and Industry Relationships: Their Impact on Medicine," *Milit. Med.* 128 (1963): 514.

39. T. B. Binns, "The Price of Therapeutic Progress," *Scot. Med. J.* 10 (1965): 130.

40. *J. Roy. Soc. Arts* 111 (1963): 856–82.

41. Tishler, "Role of the Drug House," pp. 595–96.

have, nevertheless, supplied longer accounts of this dependence of industry upon the work of others. But perhaps the best illustration of this relationship is to be found in the account of A. N. Richards,[42] one-time chairman of the Office of Scientific Research and Development Committee on Medical Research, of the work that preceded and was essential to the tremendous accomplishments of industry in the production of penicillin. This included the work of Fleming, Florey, and Chain, the development of a satisfactory culture medium by the United States Department of Agriculture, the development of better strains of the mold at the universities of Minnesota and Wisconsin, the direction and coordination of industrial activity by the OSRD, and the financial support of the War Production Board. The synthesis of penicillin, Richards also points out, took the efforts of over three hundred participants from four British and five American universities, two British and two American research foundations, one British and four American governmental agencies, and five British and ten American commercial enterprises.

In justice to our industrial spokesman, perhaps he was suggesting that an entity is not a drug until it has been processed, produced, and made available. If so, there is of course a greater validity to his statement. Without the work of Merck Sharp & Dohme in finding productive techniques, streptomycin and related antibiotics, in Waksman's own words, might have remained "bibliographic curiosities."[43] The same might well be said about the work of Eli Lilly with insulin, and probably about all the other illustrations I have used. I am aware also that not a few of the academic researches I have mentioned were supported by grants from industry. This may have been all to the good, but it hardly accounts for the years of work and experience and the accomplishments that led up to the readiness of industry to undertake assistance. I am also aware that a great deal actually did originate in industrial laboratories: the sulfa antibiotics, the diuretics, vitamin B_{12}, and the tranquilizers, to name some of the more important ones.

But if a distinction is to be made, as just suggested, between an entity and a drug, then herein lies the major significance of the pharmaceutical industry. Vast resources of scientific knowledge and engineering skills are required for the preparation, synthesis, physical production, and quality evaluation, not to mention clinical testing, of drugs. Without these resources the therapeutic revolution could never have occurred.

All of this has placed upon the industry a tremendous social obligation. The products of the industry are virtually *sui generis* and so much

42. "Production of Penicillin in the U.S. (1941–1946)," *Nature* (London) 201 (1964): 441–45.
43. "A Most Fruitful Connection," *By Their Fruits* (Rahway, N.J.: Merck Sharp & Dohme, 1962), p. 12.

more indispensable to social well-being than the ordinary commodities of the market place that the industry has found itself under close public and official scrutiny. The industry has undergone considerable criticism.[44] It is not necessary to go through the litany of abuses with which the industry has been charged, but it is significant to note that increasing involvement of government in research as well as regulation will tend to direct and limit the control which industry has heretofore exercised in the determination of which drugs are made available and of the quality of those drugs. This is not the place to pass judgment on the effect of this on public health, but it is obvious that industry will be called upon increasingly to share its responsibilities with the academic world and with government.

44. See the Kefauver Hearing Reports, the Sainsbury Report, and the Parliamentary debate on the Medicines Bill.

Commentary

Lester S. King

The three papers presented above are very different from one another. Dr. Ackerknecht has taken us on a jet-propelled survey of medical history with special reference to drug therapy, and he has restricted himself to the period before 1900. Dr. Beecher deals with the present day, and he has discussed some rather sophisticated experiments that go to the heart of what I would call the therapeutic problem: in any given situation, how do you know that a drug or medication or procedure has therapeutic effectiveness? He has shown how difficult it is to achieve a valid *measure* of psychopharmacological activity, and he has outlined his own procedure in one particular area concerned with pain. And Dr. Cowen has discussed, quite admirably, the role of industry—pharmaceutical industry—in achieving control of drug preparations.

Can we detect a common thread that runs through all of these communications? In all three papers certain words occur again and again, or, if not the identical words, at least the same basic concepts which stand behind the words. We hear about empiricism and rationalism, we hear about experiment and controls and statistics, we hear about evaluation. All of these concern the nature of scientific investigation. All of these, in my opinion, represent phases of what I would call critical acumen. To be sure, in this symposium we are talking specifically about drugs, but the problem really concerns all aspects of medical investigation. And this, I would insist, applies to the treatment of the individual patient just as much as it does to a laboratory experiment, although the conditions and circumstances are different. Medical investigation depends on what I would call critical acumen. The historians can describe the growth of critical acumen over particular time spans and contexts, while the active investigator who is not a historian can analyze his own critical methodology and the concepts behind it.

It is a great mistake to think that critical acumen had a definite beginning in time. It did not begin in the 1930's or 1940's; it did not begin with Poincaré or with Claude Bernard, or with John Stuart Mill or Pierre Louis or Magendie, or even Francis Bacon. It is the characteristic of all great physicians and investigators. I need only point to Hippocrates as a superb example of precise observation, careful reasoning, and judicious evaluation. The fact that he was utterly wrong in terms of later information and later concepts does not at all affect his critical acumen. The same remarks would apply to the much maligned Galen.

I would like to develop the concept of critical acumen, particularly in reference to medication, and I will do so largely from the historical viewpoint. If we consider, for example, the elder Pliny, we find statements about drugs that manifest a high degree of credulity. We could say he accepted claims on the basis of only hearsay evidence. But we must never make the mistake of thinking that there is no evidence. There is plenty of evidence, and the problem concerns its evaluation and acceptance. The acceptance of hearsay or tradition indicates one type of evaluation; insistence on empirical confirmation represents another. Sir Thomas Browne, by no means a model of skepticism and often noteworthy for his credulity, nevertheless demanded empirical evidence. Thus, he declared, "That Elder Berries are poison, as we are taught by tradition, experience will unteach us. And besides the promises of Blochwitius, the healthful effects thereof daily observed will convict us."

Experience alone, of course, is a weak creature which must be supported by reason. Sir Kenelm Digby, for example, had great faith in the powder of sympathy, which could work a cure without having any direct contact with the patient (he would have been quite interested in our present-day X-ray therapy). Digby not only had empirical evidence that the powder of sympathy worked, he could also explain the action by a detailed chain of events, all neatly interdigitating with each other, to furnish a sound logical basis for the alleged fact.

Obviously, direct perception alone is insufficient to establish a fact; a rational evaluation must also take place. This is perfectly clear if we attend the performance of a magician, sometimes called an illusionist, who in front of our eyes causes material objects to vanish in utter destruction and then makes them appear somewhere else. These data we do not accept as facts, despite the clear perception. The really crucial problem in empiricism concerns the question: Is a given experience a *fact*? Is a given perception, or else an assertion on "reputable" authority, a fact?

Robert Boyle was much concerned with this problem. He distinguished between what he observed with his own eyes and what others reported to have taken place. Thus, he mentioned a "very experienced and sober gentleman who is much talked of" who cured cancer of the female breast "by the outward application of an indolent powder, some of which he also gave me." But he added with deep caution that he himself had not yet had the opportunity of trying it. Clearly, as long as he could not try it himself, he withheld his judgment, no matter how experienced or sober the gentleman who reported it. Repeatedly we find him skeptical regarding claims that he himself had not verified.

But this praiseworthy sense of caution in accepting data as facts he failed to carry over into other areas where he did have direct experience. For example, he was quite convinced that millipedes, suitably prepared, were a powerful remedy, and he knew that they had great medicinal value in suffusion of the eyes—on the basis of a single case. In some clinical trials he dealt with large numbers of patients; in one experiment wherein he followed Van Helmont's techniques, but with improvements, he made a purified medicine that he found to be "a potent specifick for the rickets," and he asserted that he "cured" a hundred or more children of that disease.

We say immediately that he had no controls. Yet Boyle was a top-notch scientist. He had good judgment and sharp critical acumen. The significant point about his clinical experiments was not that he lacked controls but that he did not perceive the need for controls. Boyle, in the 1660's, was the most prominent member of the Royal Society, which was founded on the precepts of Francis Bacon. Bacon had indicated the need for controlled experiments; nevertheless, Boyle, the leading scientist of the Society, found complete conviction in his experience, without the use of controls. This is not in any way a condemnation of Boyle, or a condemnation of the seventeenth century. It is a commentary on the growth of critical attitudes.

If we jump forward into the latter eighteenth century and the first part of the nineteenth, we find a rather different situation. Samuel Hahnemann, the founder of homeopathy, exhibited a quite different kind of attitude. We tend to forget that Hahnemann was an experimental pharmacologist who conducted studies in psychopharmacology and tried to identify the reactions that various therapeutic substances produced in consciousness. He began his experimental career in 1790, when he deliberately dosed himself with quinine and found that he had symptoms that simulated fever—all symptoms, that is, except the "actual febrile rigor." We remember, of course, that the physician in those days had quite different criteria for identifying fever than he has today.

He himself served as a normal healthy subject. Every time he took quinine he had the same symptoms, which passed off when the drug was not taken. Thus he served as his own control, and he could correlate symptoms with the experimental procedure, absence of symptoms with the periods of rest. This was reasonably good planning, but unfortunately he generalized widely on his series of one case. On the basis of his own experience alone, he drew the conclusion that a medicinal substance can induce a disease. Quinine, which cured fever, could itself produce "fever." Or at least it produced the symptoms which Hahnemann *called* fever.

He also performed other pharmacological experiments to determine the effect of various medicinal substances on normal healthy humans.

His technique, however, had certain great flaws, for the indicator of medicinal action depended solely on introspection. He assumed that an observer, by describing his own state of consciousness, can identify and describe all the physiological actions of the substance taken. He ignored any effect that did not appear in consciousness. Furthermore, he assumed that, after the taking of a drug, everything that could be introspected was the result of that drug. I have discussed these errors more fully elsewhere.

Hahnemann's doctrines, as they developed over more than a quarter of a century, form a fascinating study in methodology. His conception of a "fact" was limited, and his mind was closed to evidence that ran contrary to his doctrines. He simply ignored what did not fit. It is hard to justify such an attitude, especially when better examples were available to him, such as that of James Lind.

Hahnemann, we would say, lacked critical acumen. I cannot at this time enter into a precise definition of this concept, but I would indicate at least one component—the awareness that maybe the entity in question, whatever it is we are investigating, does not exist. The supposed fact may actually be an error; the particular inference may be incorrect. Or, as Oliver Cromwell so expertly phrased it, "By the bowels of Christ I beseech ye, bethink yourselves that ye may be mistaken." If we do bethink ourselves of this, we are well on the way to critical acumen. This implies humility, which Boyle possessed to a high degree, but which was quite lacking in Hahnemann.

The question "What *is* a fact?" assumed new prominence with Pierre Louis and his well known numerical method, with its emphasis on controls. In one of his best known papers, Louis directed his method to the study of bloodletting. His critical observations helped to impair the faith in that therapy, faith that had lasted for millennia and yet crumbled in less than a generation. I would like to emphasize, however, that Louis' conclusions, derived from his statistical analysis, are not valid according to present-day thought.

It is not results that are important, however, but the attitude toward evidence. This attitude, which I call critical acumen, is the indispensable weapon of the investigator or the good clinician. It has developed slowly over the past three or four centuries, forging for itself various helpful tools. Neither the numerical method of Louis nor the double-blind experiment of today comprise, of themselves, the critical attitude. They are only tools, comparable, perhaps, to Francis Bacon's tables of similarity and tables of difference. Bacon thought his tabulation and comparison would constitute a method that could place all wits on a level. It did nothing of the sort, of course. The essential feature that Bacon left out of account was the flash of intuition that could not be placed in a table, the intuition that the perceptive man has and the dullard does not have.

Similarly, double-blind techniques do not place all wits on a level but serve only as instruments.

The study of drugs has been one of the most important areas in the slow painful growth of critical acumen. And this aspect of scientific methodology has been, I believe, a common thread through all these contributions.

Commentary

Karl H. Beyer, Jr.

My own creed, the quotation by which I live and for which many of you in this room can cite the source, is that "Science progresses by successive approximations to the truth." It is a good creed. It is a hopeful one, on the one hand, and on the other it reminds me that nothing I do in research will be entirely right or adequate, at least from the standpoint of interpretation. The whole thread of history pretty much bears this out: there have been so many aspects of medicine which seemed to be real and substantial at the moment, but which have given way as the cumulative evidence of time has provided a more adequate basis for judgment.

In many respects, the themes of medical history obtain today. Others have spoken here of the authoritarian aspects of medicine in a historical setting, yet they are very real today. They are very real at a national level, where, for example, physicians in Sweden look first to their Swedish literature to establish for them the credibility of a new therapeutic agent, and the same may be said of men in any other country. In this country and abroad, even at a local level, one or two physicians will be found who are the leaders in a field and to whom others look for what is proper in medicine, what is a good drug that is safe or useful. These authoritarian influences derive from clinical experience in part, just as they have throughout the history of medicine.

The empiricisms of today, in the sense in which the authors have used the term, relate to the differences in concept of what constitutes adequate clinical investigation. In this country, a fixed double-blind study is preferred to the open-ended sequential analysis that finds favor in England.

There still remains a demoniac aspect of modern medicine, which I had to learn a few years ago when we introduced into clinical study a new anticholinergic agent. Its virtue, we felt from the laboratory data, was that it should not produce substantial effects on other than the upper gastrointestinal anticholinergic target, which was our objective. It was really impossible, or so it turned out, to get a good study of this seeming virtue. The physician was so used to the blurring of vision, the dryness of mouth, and the retention of urine induced by anticholinergic drugs that he simply would not study the compound at dosages where it did not produce these familiar side effects.

The history of medicine gives strong basis for the need of leaders to maintain an open mind with respect to what is good or adequate in concept or methodology in medical research. Dr. Ackerknecht referred to Withering as an astute clinician not trained, or inclined, perhaps, to the controlled study and yet quite capable of discerning a useful therapy when it was available to him. Dr. Ackerknecht also referred to Withering's contemporary in Vienna, Stoerck, who had a reasonable and even almost modern approach to the controlled study; yet he seemed utterly unable to arrive at a valid conclusion.

Dr. Beecher referred to what he called contrived pain, and to pathological pain, and to the time and effort it took men expert in this field to discern their difference. As I read his manuscript I wondered about the course of medical history if morphine and saline had not been found statistically different in the contrived human double-blind test and if we did not have the historical background of experience with morphine as an analgesic agent. I think the results would have been negative, as he indicated. The literature would recite the elegant experiments from which the deduction was reached that morphine and saline were *not* different. Only time and more appropriate experiments could be counted on to right the record. Dr. Beecher's experience recites in modern terms the history of drug experimentation. Thus, quite apart from the experimental design, quite apart from the statistical analysis—all of which we have today in complex elegance—is the need for appropriateness of the experiment to the clinical situation, if the results are to be helpful.

The history of medicine recites the importance of adequate control of purity and uniformity. This need brought biologists into the industrial laboratories to assure product uniformity by bioassay. Sometimes what was done was, unwittingly, inadequate to assure the safety and uniformity of a new product. Dr. Cowen referred to the early difficulties with the new diphtheria antitoxin when it was first made available. It had to be removed for further investigation before its safety was established. One does not have to go back to diphtheria antitoxin for an analogy. The problems that related to the inactivation of polio vaccine are recent history. The approved procedure for its inactivation needed to be made more reliable to assure that no live polio virus remained in the product. As one works within the limits of knowledge to create new therapy as a service to mankind, one is confronted by these realities. Regardless of who excercises product control in such matters from a regulatory standpoint, it is the company and finally its personnel who expose themselves to, and sometimes live with, tragedy.

Medicine, pharmacy, and the drug industry are all much older than research in the industry. The history of medicine vividly contrasts the progress made in therapy since research was brought "in house" in the pharmaceutical industry with what had developed before that time. This does not mean that the industry can take credit for this progress, but it is proud to have shared in it. There is always room for controversy among groups and individuals as to where credit is most due, but our progress has been great enough so that we can all derive satisfaction from it. Furthermore, it is clear that the advances in therapy have been greatest in countries where the motivation is most adequate.

In closing these remarks I should add that I am not a historian: I work today and for tomorrow, and yet one intuitively looks to the past to anticipate the alternatives that the future may present. This is an exciting and serious time in medical history. How well we do sustain national resources of government, university, and industry to assure our recent rate of productivity for the greatest common good is the larger issue to which we address ourselves as we look to the past for guidance.

Discussion

Dr. Blake: Thank you, Dr. Beyer. I would now like to call for comments from the floor.

Mr. Janssen: With regard to the history of the pharmaceutical industry, I think it is important not to neglect the impact of major wars. The Civil War, for example, greatly stimulated the development of the American pharmaceutical industry, which hardly existed before 1861. Both sides were unable to get sufficient supplies of drugs, and the ones they could get often were provided by incompetent or even dishonest contractors and were very unsatisfactory. Both sides set up production facilities, but the federal government in particular developed mass production facilities at Brooklyn and Philadelphia. An important byproduct of this was the training of pharmaceutical manufacturing personnel. I believe a young medical officer named Squibb was the commander of the Brooklyn laboratory. It was this war experience that really started the pharmaceutical industry in the United States as we know it today.

In World War II the government took a different approach to the problem of securing sufficient supplies—particularly and specifically of the important drug penicillin, which was desperately needed on the battlefield. Instead of engaging in production, the government put large sums of money into stimulating the pharmaceutical industry to expand production quickly. There was a "crash" program to get penicillin as fast as possible. Penicillin production and a couple of very secret projects, the atom bomb and the proximity fuse, were the three big scientific production efforts in World War II.

Dr. Benison: I would like to underline something that Dr. King said about the nature of scientific investigation, because I think it had much point. When Dubos analyzes the work of his chief, the famous O. T. Avery, he says that, of all the men he knew in science, Avery was the least addicted to experimentation. Rather, he was concerned with defining the architecture of the problem and redefining it, not by experimentation, but by conversation. Of course, he had magnificent conversation in that laboratory.

I would also like to open up a Pandora's box which the panel has thus far avoided, namely, the problem of the ethics of experimentation, because eventually it comes down to human experimentation.

Dr. Beyer: It would be hard for me to envision going from laboratory research, even in primates, directly to clinical trial with any drug. When I say "directly" and "primates," I do this deliberately, because in my experience—or more properly in the experience of those in my laboratory —the metabolic variation between primates is as great in many instances as it is between primates and other animals. To my way of thinking, for progress there is no recourse other than to clinical study.

Dr. Ackerknecht: I think that those who oppose the controlled clinical trial are wrong, that there is no way of replacing or avoiding this.

I might add that this ethical question perhaps explains the frequent self-experiments. People themselves had the feeling that human experiments were ethically rather doubtful, and to justify them they inserted the self-experiment between the animal experiment and the clinical trial. It is surprising on what scale self-experiment has been used.

Dr. Beyer: I think we have all done this and felt morally that this was right, that if we took it first, this was fine. The Nuremberg code, of course, recognized that this is specious reasoning, and I think rightly. The fact that one is sufficiently foolhardy to take a new compound without adequate assessment gives him no license to try it on his neighbor.

Dr. King: In continuation of that subject, we may note that investigators sometimes insert themselves first, in the trial of a drug, and then they insert members of their family, which is sort of a next step, and then they try it out on somebody else.

If we are going to get into this question, however, we might as well get in with both feet and see where the path goes. The problem of ethics of drug trials has, it seems to me, a strong parallel with the problems of the financial exploitation of drugs. We all know that there have been great abuses, and we blame these on the venality of manufacturers and business-men in general. We who are in pure science are much above this sort of venality, and we think we can look down our noses at those people who have to deal with the dollar. But in research there may be a comparable type of exploitation of the public. With the tremendous amount of highly subsidized research going on, we now have a large class of researchers who, to get ahead in the world of research, must do a lot of clinical experimentation. Consequently, I think the ethical sensibilities of many of our researchers are somewhat blunted, in a manner analogous to the way the ethical sensibilities of some business men are blunted when they try to market their product in the face of strong competition. I think that a great many morally and ethically unjustifiable experiments are being undertaken in order to get ahead in the academic world. This is, of course, my personal reaction.

Dr. Lasagna: In regard to the ethics of drug development and clinical test-ing, one might observe that if we are engaged in a war we do not randomly put into the "pot" all the males in the country, including congressmen, the President, and so forth, pull them out at random, and send them off to the battlefields. We are quite arbitrary in what we do, usually in the interest of what we call the "greater good." I think that there is on many occasions an irreconcilable conflict between the interest of the individual patient and the interest of scientific progress, as in the development of remedies that will perhaps in the long run help a great many people. This does not make the individual experiment any easier to deal with ethically. Each situation has to be dealt with on its own merits and each person has to sleep with his own conscience, as well as with his worries about what the lawyers may do to him. But I do think it is a problem that society has not paid enough attention to.

Mr. Cowen: In regard to the draft, I do not like the word "arbitrary." These actions are done by due process of law, and this is not exactly arbitrary. The same thing might be said with regard to ethics in medicine; there can be, and may even have been, some attempt to deal with these problems in advance and not necessarily arbitrarily.

★ ★ ★ ★ ★

Dr. Blake: At this time I would like to offer the original speakers an opportunity to make further comments.

Dr. Ackerknecht: I enjoyed Dr. King's remarks very much. He introduced the "critical acumen." That comes pretty close to the genius of Zimmermann, but Dr. King made a better argument for it, and he did something, he introduced the tools for the critical acumen, which Zimmermann mostly left out. Now, I must confess quite frankly I myself feel there is something to this critical acumen—that is why I brought in Withering; it is not just the tools. On the other hand, I feel that real critical acumen is so rare that we must—and I think that this has been the course of history—invent as many tools as possible. They are still incomplete and new ones have to be invented—and will be invented—to enable the individual who is not gifted with great critical acumen to handle these problems. In our mass society, this is even less avoidable than before.

Dr. King: I want to make one small explanatory comment. Perhaps the major difference between Dr. Ackerknecht and myself is that he applies the concept of critical acumen (assuming we agree on it) to those experiments which are successful and which have resulted in positive benefits that are still demonstrable today, whereas I feel that the concept of critical acumen may be appropriately applied to workers who were absolutely wrong. They could still demonstrate what I would call critical acumen, even in being wrong.

Part III: Private Professional Controls

Contribution of the Pharmaceutical Profession Toward Controlling the Quality of Drugs in the Nineteenth Century

Glenn Sonnedecker

An element of control over the quality of drugs, in a broad sense, pervades the classical functions of pharmacy as a specialized service within a responsible system of medical care. The pharmacist feels this most forcefully as compounder and dispenser of medicines, but it extends to all those functions in a textbook definition of pharmacy that includes "identification, selection, preservation, combination, analysis, and standardization" of medicinal substances.[1] To avoid complication, we shall speak here of the "pharmaceutical profession" as though it included all those persons and institutions whose purposes were primarily pharmaceutical. In speaking of the "pharmacist," we shall mean only someone qualified to practice pharmacy.[2]

This discussion will be divided into two parts by the year 1865: after the Civil War both the social and scientific means of control over the quality of drugs changed more rapidly and reached a distinctively different level of maturity. Each period will be examined briefly for the relevance to drug quality of three central developments: self-control, legal control, and technical specifications.

Before 1865

Role of Self-Control. Belief in voluntary control and free competition dominated efforts to assure the quality of drugs—and of pharmaceutical services generally—in the period before the Civil War. The pharmacists' contribution toward controlling quality was fashioned largely by a minority who knew at first or second hand the traditions and literature of pharmacy abroad, especially in England, France, or Germany, and who wanted the title of apothecary and druggist to merit respect as well as money.

1. E. F. Cook and E. W. Martin, eds., *Remington's Practice of Pharmacy*, 10th ed. (Easton, Pa.: Mack, 1951), p. 1.
2. Until after the Civil War, the usual term for a public practitioner of pharmacy was "pharmaceutist" or "apothecary." The term "druggist" ordinarily implied a wholesale druggist, whose operations might include to some extent both manufacturing and dispensing; but by the 1880's the unmodified term "druggist" was well on its way toward becoming synonymous with a newly popular term, "pharmacist."

This paper was prepared while the writer held a University of Wisconsin research appointment under a grant from the United States Pharmacopeial Convention.

Their initiative was repeatedly spurred by physicians concerned with the quality of therapeutic agents they no longer found it feasible to prepare and dispense themselves. Their effectiveness depended substantially upon the development of a pharmaceutical service that would be more of a protection than a risk, more of a profession than a business.[3]

The first organized move came from the pharmacists who founded and operated the seven local associations, called colleges, which had been formed by 1865. All but two promptly established schools of pharmacy.[4] The first and strongest, the Philadelphia College of Pharmacy (founded 1821), illustrates the concern with controlling drug quality. The writers of the college's constitution viewed with alarm the varying methods in use for preparing the same drug, the varying strengths under the same name, and the difficulty of detecting many adulterations of drugs, all of which, they declared, "offer great incitements to cupidity and open a wide door to abuses. . . ." In a gesture bold for the time, the Constitution provided for expulsion of any member "guilty of adulterating or sophisticating any articles of medicine or drugs, or of knowingly vending articles of that character. . . ." The bylaws set up a five-man Committee of Inspection to examine drugs submitted to them and to report to the board "such unmerchantable or spurious Drugs and Medicines as may come within their knowledge."[5]

Indeed, it was reportedly a case of fraudulent opium purchased by one of the principal Philadelphia druggists that "first impressed the apothecaries and druggists of Philadelphia with the necessity of exercising some supervision over the sale of medicines."[6] In the America of the 1820's, this "supervision" implied group self-discipline rather than government intervention.

When was it justifiable to impose demands beyond a person's own conscience? Although spokesmen for the College would differ somewhat in different decades when discussing that question, in the 1820's it was logical to find "The genius of our political institutions, precluding the

3. For evidences of the trend toward the separation of pharmacy and medicine, see *The Pharmacopoeia of the Massachusetts Medical Society* (Boston: E. & J. Larkin, 1808), p. v; "Introduction," *J. Phila. Coll. Pharm.* 1 (1826): 1; W. R. Fisher, "A Brief Sketch of the Progress and Present State of Pharmacy in the United States of America," *Amer. J. Pharm.* n.s. 2 (1837): 271–79.

4. All pharmacist-sponsored associations were located in the northeast. The only nonassociation school during this period was a pharmacy department within the Medical School of Tulane University, at New Orleans.

5. *The Constitution and By-laws of the College of Apothecaries of Philadelphia* (Philadelphia, 1821), pp. 3, 16. A Committee of Inspection was utilized by the College at least occasionally to curb drug adulteration (see Minute Book of the Philadelphia College of Apothecaries, No. 1, March 25, 1823; unpaginated MS. in Registrar's Office, Philadelphia College of Pharmacy and Science).

6. Daniel B. Smith, "Address Delivered by the President . . . [at] Commencement," *J. Phila. Coll. Pharm.* n.s. 1 (1830): 256.

introduction of the European system, for the regulation of pharmacy. . . ." Yet the College recognized "That the sale and dispensation of drugs and medicines, are liable to abuses from ignorance or design; that serious dangers threaten society from this cause; and that countervailing measures are, consequently, requisite. . . ."[7] In view of sporadic complaints about "spurious and inert medicines," the College Secretary wrote in the minutes, "It is certain that the honour of the College requires that this subject must sooner or later engage its attention &, that this heinous offence against morality & justice should not remain a reproachful stain upon the character of [pharmacy]. . . ."[8]

The New York College of Pharmacy—founded eight years after that in Philadelphia—likewise spoke of the "evil" of substandard drugs that existed "to a very alarming extent." Its members found tartaric acid that was half alum, ipecac that was adulterated with sarsaparilla, morphine acetate that was wholly calcium sulfate, volatile oils that were cut with cheaper ones.[9] The New York College maintained an active Committee of Inspection modeled after the one at the Philadelphia College and published a series of reports on samples of adulterated drugs analyzed, the methods applicable, and sometimes the names of houses where substandard drugs were purchased.[10]

In each of the colleges of pharmacy before 1865 there would have been at least a few pharmaceutists or faculty members who could apply to market samples the quality tests then commonly known. Moreover, the *Pharmacopoeia of the United States* current in 1865 still listed only a few drugs with specifications going beyond crude organoleptic and flame or solubility tests. Such tests could be applied by an experienced and conscientious pharmaceutist, even if he was meagerly educated. The most important control on quality he was expected to exercise, however, was to choose his crude or raw drugs carefully and prepare his medications skillfully by the formula and process specified in the *Pharmacopoeia*, or, when there was need, another authoritative guide.

Reaching a wider audience than meetings of the seven colleges, the *American Journal of Pharmacy* began publication in 1825[11] as the first professional scientific journal of its kind in English. It was one of the

7. *The Charter, Regulations, and By-laws, of the Philadelphia College of Pharmacy* (Philadelphia: S. W. Conrad, 1826), pp. i–ii.

8. Minute Book, No. 1, Dec. 31, 1822.

9. Oliver Hull, "On Adulterations of Certain Medicines," *Amer. J. Pharm.* n.s. 1 (1835): 11; see also W. L. Rushton, "Extract from a Communication . . . on the Adulteration of Medicines," *Amer. J. Pharm.* n.s. 1 (1835): 30.

10. Curt P. Wimmer, *The College of Pharmacy of the City of New York* (Baltimore: Read-Taylor, 1929), pp. 192–96.

11. Known until 1835 as the *Journal of the Philadelphia College of Pharmacy*. Still published by that College, it is now the oldest English-language journal of pharmacy in continuous publication.

most constructive and consistent forces of the nineteenth century for improving the quality of drugs. Especially before 1865, the *Journal* set new goals more than it reflected what could be expected of the average American drug dispenser.

The cultivation of a spirit of identity, emulation, and responsibility among members of the few local societies of pharmaceutists and druggists generated most of the aspiration that led to the founding of the American Pharmaceutical Association in 1852. Reacting against the political emasculation of the first national law designed to control the quality of drug imports, the New York College of Pharmacy had called a meeting of the colleges of pharmacy in October, 1851, to consider "the propriety and practicability of fixing a set of standard strengths and qualities of drugs and chemicals for the government of the United States Drug Inspectors."[12] This led to a meeting with more general aims in 1852, where the national society was organized. In a strikingly analogous way, just five years earlier, the New York State Medical Society had called a meeting for the purpose of a limited reform which led to broader aims and, a year later, to the founding of the American Medical Association.[13] It is significant that the Constitution of the Pharmaceutical Association stated first among its objects: "To improve and regulate the drug market, by preventing the importation of inferior, adulterated or deteriorated drugs, and by detecting and exposing home adulteration."

Thus, before the Civil War, a foundation had been laid for a group consciousness and conscience in pharmacy and for a system of pharmaceutical education. A responsible class had emerged which later legislation could hold accountable as part of a publicly authorized and controlled system of medical care.

Role of Compulsory Control. Although spotty and ineffectual, even before 1865 legislation began to establish principles and patterns for better controls over the quality of drugs. Efforts were made to certify competence and control practice through a licensing system and to make intentional debasement of drugs illegal. Modest controls over the practice of pharmacy were adopted before the Civil War in four states, all in the South, as part of broader plans to regulate the practice of medicine. There were in addition a few local laws specifically related to the practice of pharmacy, but they were mostly considered ineffectual.[14]

12. *Amer. J. Pharm.* 24 (1852): 86.
13. Wimmer, *The College of Pharmacy*, p. 204; Richard H. Shryock, *Medical Licensing in America* (Baltimore: Johns Hopkins Press, 1967), pp. 28–33. On the Import Act of 1848, see below p. 101-2.
14. Glenn Sonnedecker, *Kremers and Urdang's History of Pharmacy*, 3d ed. (Philadelphia: Lippincott, 1963), pp. 193–95. Fisher, "A Brief Sketch," *Amer. J. Pharm.* n.s. 2 (1837): 274. The states were Louisiana, South Carolina, Georgia, and Alabama; the cities were New Orleans, La., New York, N.Y., Natchez, Miss., and Louisville, Ky.

The hesitant development of pharmaceutical licensure in part reflected the circumstance of medicine at the time. Just when pharmacy was developing sufficient organization and a system of education to permit it to emulate medicine, the licensing system of its sister profession was itself deteriorating. While the reasons are complex, negative influences included proprietary medical schools, attacks from medical sects (botanic, and homeopathic), and Americans' distrust of anything that might threaten freedom or encourage monopoly.[15]

Early legislation that in some way attempted to deal with drug adulteration was adopted by at least fourteen states before 1865.[16] However, efforts to prosecute frequently faced the almost insurmountable handicap of having to prove willful or fraudulent adulteration of drugs in a manner injurious to health. If such laws designated an enforcement agency, the supporting appropriation, if any, was ordinarily meager.[17] The deterrent effect could scarcely have been oppressive for that unknown number of unprincipled drug dealers who were intent upon deception.

Moreover, even conscientious druggists and pharmaceutists could not always safeguard the prescribing physician and his patients from cleverly debased drugs. Responsible pharmaceutists became especially concerned about the adulteration of imports, which the United States depended upon before the Civil War for most of its raw drugs and intermediate products. This culminated in one of the most important events of the nineteenth century within the scope of our present concern, congressional enactment in 1848 of a national drug-import law.

The College of Pharmacy of the City of New York, which had taken the initiative in this matter, passed a resolution pledging "all proper measures to expose" drug adulterators and help "make this salutary law effective."[18] The act was thus inaugurated with high hopes, and in the first ten months 90,000 pounds of drugs were turned back at the port of

15. See Shryock, *Medical Licensing in America*, pp. 28–33.
16. Representative early legislative provisions were those of Louisiana (1808), Massachusetts (1836), Vermont (1839), and Rhode Island (1844). For information on the extent of early enactments, I am indebted to Professor David L. Cowen of Rutgers, The State University of New Jersey.
17. Vermont (1839) penalized "fraudulently adulterating for sale . . . drug or medicine so as to render it injurious" (*Revised Statutes*, p. 445); Rhode Island (1844) penalized "fraudulently adulterating for the purpose of sale, any drug or medicine, in such a manner as to render the same injurious to health" (*R. I. Laws*, Sec. 111, p. 397); while Tennessee (before 1858) referred to adulteration that would "lessen the efficacy or change the operation injurious to health" (*Code of Tennessee*, 1858, p. 865).
18. Wimmer, *The College of Pharmacy*, pp. 199–200; and, on the College's wider concern and controversies relating to drug quality, pp. 192–204; on the role of the Philadelphia College and its Committee on Adulteration of Drugs, see its Minutes, No. 2, June 30, 1847, and Nov. 1, 1847 (MS. in Registrar's Office, Philadelphia College of Pharmacy and Science).

entry.[19] Enforcement was based upon an examination at the customhouse of medicinally intended substances "as well in reference to their quality, purity, and fitness for medicinal purposes, as to their value and identity specified in the invoice." The basis of judgment was inferiority "in strength and purity to the standard established by the United States, Edinburgh, London, French and German pharmacopoeias and dispensatories, and thereby improper. . . ." To help carry out this check, the Secretary of the Treasury was directed "to appoint suitably qualified persons as special examiners" at principal ports of entry.[20]

Sanguine expectations were dissipated when it became clear what an enormous range of specification and judgment was permitted by the diverse pharmacopoeias and dispensatories of five countries. Moreover, it was charged, and apparently proved, that the elasticity in enforcing the 1848 act was aggravated by federal drug examiners who had been appointed more for their political influence than for their technical competence. In addition, experience with the law brought new awareness that all drug adulterators were not foreigners, as it had been tempting for some to assume. The *American Journal of Pharmacy* reluctantly concluded that the 1848 enactment would prove to be only the first step in "necessary reforms of a monstrous evil."[21]

Role of Specifications. To meet the problem head-on required an adequate definition of acceptable quality for each drug. This meant technical specifications or standards by which those with professional competence could judge shipments of a drug that came to hand. Then as now, the central goal was therapeutic equivalency for all drugs used in medical care under the same name. The degree of equivalency, of course, could never surpass the level of science and technology that could be brought to bear at a particular time.

The physician hoped for a uniformity permitting confidence that from one prescription to the next there would be no difference of significance to the patient in the effects of a drug. Most civilized countries relied primarily on a national pharmacopoeia, that is, a compilation of specifications for drugs designed to bring about uniformity of composition, strength, and purity, adapted to the needs of a particular political unit, acceptable to representatives of the medical profession, and made obligatory for all those responsible for the supply of drugs.[22]

19. "Adulteration of Drugs," *Amer. J. Pharm.* n.s. 15 (1849): 382–83; see also pp. 153–69.
20. Wimmer, *The College of Pharmacy*, pp. 196, 199.
21. "Adulteration of Drugs," *Amer. J. Pharm.* n.s. 15 (1849): 382–84; Wimmer, *The College of Pharmacy*, pp. 202–4.
22. George Urdang, "Pharmacopoeias as Witnesses of World History," *J. Hist. Med.* 1 (1946): 46.

For such standards to be effective or obligatory requires enforcement. The *Pharmacopoeia of the United States* lacked legal authority during this period and during the rest of the century in most "political units" of the country. Such authority could not be conveyed by any volunteer effort of physicians and pharmacists or by state laws requiring proof of "adulteration" that was intentional and harmful to the patient.

The constructive effect of the U.S. *Pharmacopoeia*, first issued in December, 1820, is clear, yet extremely difficult to evaluate. Commonly called "official" as a mark of respect, it carried only the collective authority of the medical institutions whose representatives brought it into being. These delegates convened every ten years, on a democratic basis, as the National Medical Convention. Since no counterpart institutions of pharmacists existed in 1820, the participation of pharmacists in creating the *Pharmacopoeia* was not an issue, but it was recognized that their cooperation was essential to make it effective.[23]

Having relied on voluntary work and democratic decision-making for the creation of the *Pharmacopoeia*, organized medicine, and later organized pharmacy, also relied on voluntary compliance. It thus seemed a characteristic American venture of free and independent professions.

The first *Pharmacopoeia* consisted of two parts: a list of the materia medica, including chemical compounds, crude drugs, fixed oils, and other substances kept by the apothecary, though generally prepared elsewhere; and a formulary of compositions to be made by the apothecary alone. This basic structure continued until the latter part of the century.

From the first to the sixth decennial revision, the College of Physicians of Philadelphia was the center for the scientific work. It developed a spirit of emulation and cooperation with the Philadelphia College of Pharmacy. The first harbinger was experimental work on certain pharmacopoeial drugs done by the President of the Philadelphia College of Pharmacy, Daniel B. Smith,[24] who later became the first president of the American Pharmaceutical Association.

"We must possess a Pharmacopoeia," Smith had said, "adapted to the condition of this country, and founded upon strict analysis and experiment . . . without blindly following the formulae of any foreign college. . . ."[25] The Revision Committee for the 1831 edition attributed

23. *Pharmacopoeia of the United States of America* (Boston: Wells and Lilly, 1820), p. 7.
24. See "DBS" and "EE" to G. B. Wood, 3 pp. (n.p., n.d. [ca. 1830]), in "Reports of the Committee of the College of Physicians on the Revision of the Pharmacopoeia," unbound manuscripts at 10a/125 in College of Physicians of Philadelphia Library.
25. D. B. Smith, "Address Delivered by the President," *J. Phila. Coll. Pharm.* n.s. 1 (1830): 244. On Smith, see Joseph W. England, ed., *The First Century of the Philadelphia College of Pharmacy, 1821–1921* (Philadelphia: Philadelphia College of Pharmacy and Science, 1922), pp. 353–54.

deficiencies in the preceding edition to "the comparative backwardness of pharmacy in this country"; yet the editors indicated that the National Medical Convention "evinced a due regard to the progressive state of pharmaceutic science, and a laudable distrust of the adequacy of their own labours in the arduous undertaking in which they had engaged." They pointedly stated that one requirement of definitive work on standards was "a thorough acquaintance with the subject of pharmacy in all its details. . . ."[26] They submitted the final draft of the 1831 edition to the College of Pharmacy for examination; the College approved it and urged its members "to use the formulae thereof in their pharmaceutical preparations."[27]

At the Pharmacopoeial Convention in 1840, the Committee was authorized "to request the co-operation of Colleges of Pharmacy," and the groups at Philadelphia, Boston, and New York all helped to formulate standards for drugs in the 1842 edition. The Philadelphians prepared a revision of the entire *Pharmacopoeia*. Their collaboration was taken seriously enough by the physicians constituting the Revision Committee for them to delay publication about a year and wholly rewrite the work.[28]

One of the most significant changes, from the viewpoint of controlling the quality of drugs, was what the Revision Committee described as "the introduction, in connexion with certain articles of the Materia Medica and certain Preparations, of brief notes indicating the readiest means of ascertaining their genuineness and purity."[29] This refers to tests for specific gravity and solubility, and simple tests of qualitative analysis. The U.S. *Pharmacopoeia* took its cue from the London and Edinburgh pharmacopoeias, which had added similar tests in editions then current. In the two subsequent revisions before 1865, such tests were elaborated for some drugs and added to specifications for others, without a major change in the character of the drug standardization program.

Leading pharmacists also continued to conduct experimental work and otherwise improve the specifications for U.S.P. drugs. Moreover, at the 1850 Decennial Convention, five pharmacists participated as delegates and two were made members of the Committee of Revision. At the 1860 Convention, eleven pharmacists participated from four colleges of pharmacy along the eastern seaboard and half of the Revision Committee

26. *Pharmacopoeia* (1831), p. xiii.
27. *Ibid.*, p. xi.
28. *Pharmacopoeia* (1842), pp. vii–xii; "Report of the Committee of Revision of the Philadelphia College of Pharmacy on the United States Pharmacopoeia 1840," 2 vols., 357 leaves + 42 leaves, bound with Minutes of the Committee; MS. in Dean's Office, Philadelphia College of Pharmacy and Science. See also Records of the College of Physicians of Philadelphia, vols. 2 and 3, in the College Library; see entries Dec. 24, 1839, and March 3, 1840. Pharmacists William Procter, Jr., and William Hodgson, Jr., undertook extensive experimental work.
29. *Pharmacopoeia* (1842), p. xvii.

were pharmacists. The American Pharmaceutical Association—founded just eight years before—contributed a compilation of technical material.[30]

With these changes, the term National Medical Convention became obsolete, and the 1863 edition was issued "By Authority of the National Convention for Revising the Pharmacopoeia." While this signified pharmacy's full partnership in conducting the *Pharmacopoeia*, it also stimulated further development within pharmacy. Said William Fisher:

> The invitation . . . to participate . . . renders still more imperative upon us the duty of qualifying our students so that they may be competent to partake of these [pharmacopoeial] deliberations, and aid in that research which is to provide a code for the conduct of the entire profession. . . . A no more honorable motive to exertion, or more commendable ambition can well be excited, than that which is thus held out of the opportunity for a seat in that council which is to legislate [drug standards] for the whole nation.[31]

Even though Fisher used the term "legislate" in a metaphorical sense, his remark does imply the high respect and enthusiasm accorded to the pharmacopoeial program.

With no system of compulsory licensing except in a few localities, and with no formal education required, the average drug dispenser before 1865 was poorly equipped either to make or to test drugs at the level seen as a goal by the knowledgeable pharmacists associated with the *Pharmacopoeia* and with the college faculties. Yet foundations had been laid that after the Civil War transformed the pharmaceutical resources for controlling the quality of drugs.

After 1865

Role of Self-Control. Most pharmacists interested in improving the control of drug quality found a medium in the state pharmaceutical associations, most of which were established with encouragement from the American Pharmaceutical Association during the last third of the century. While most of them functioned like ordinary trade associations, a number maintained committees on drug adulteration to check drug samples and to publicize information and methods that might help safeguard against substandard drugs.[32] The American Pharmaceutical Association also had such a Committee on Adulteration for many years, and its *Proceedings* throughout the second half of the nineteenth century testify to a concern with improving the dependability of drugs. By the late nineteenth century professionally ambitious members would agree

30. See *Proc. Amer. Pharm. Ass.* 8 (1859): 217–45.
31. William Fisher, "Introductory Lecture," *Amer. J. Pharm.* 8 (1843): 12.
32. See *Proc. Penn. Pharm. Ass.*, 1892, pp. 39ff.; 1894, pp. 58–62; 1896, p. 80.

each year to investigate some pharmaceutical question raised at the meeting and to report their findings at a subsequent meeting.[33]

Leading pharmacists also became active after the Civil War in expanding the number and quality of pharmacy schools. Most significant was the establishment of pharmacy departments within state universities, especially in the Midwest. The first one was authorized at the University of Michigan in 1868; its director perfected the earliest quantitative assays specified by the U.S. *Pharmacopoeia*.[34]

At the end of the century the first Ph.D. candidate in pharmacy—at the University of Wisconsin—held a research fellowship of the United States Pharmacopoeia and was "expected to conduct research in the line of revision of the Pharmacopoeia. . . ."[35] As other universities followed Wisconsin's lead, graduate programs raised to a higher level the development of technical specification tests for the quality of drugs. During the last quarter of the century the better schools of pharmacy also began to put undergraduates into laboratories where they learned to apply chemical and microscopical procedures.

Such students were in the minority, however, since no state required formal pharmaceutical education to qualify for the licensing examinations which were being widely adopted during the last third of the century.[36] Thus it is doubtful that the average practicing pharmacist in America ever routinely applied pharmacopoeial tests to the medications that he dispensed. Yet the pharmacist exercised a scientific sense of responsibility as the last link in a chain of medicopharmacal services and the guarantor that the patient would receive exactly what was intended, in the form and quality intended. This function was of no small consequence, especially before passage of the federal Food and Drug Act (1906).

Role of Compulsory Control. By 1870 at least twenty-five states and territories had some statutory provision on drug adulteration.[37] This effort was subsequently extended and somewhat strengthened through the influence of a model pharmacy bill sponsored by the American Pharmaceutical Association. Statutes similar to it were adopted in about thirty-two states by 1890, and in another thirteen by the end of the

33. See the thirty-seven pharmaceutical questions raised and assigned by the Committee on Queries, *Proc. Amer. Pharm. Ass.* 18 (1870): 58–62.
34. Professor Albert B. Prescott, M.D., of the University of Michigan, offered processes for opium and its preparations, for cinchona bark, and for strychnine. Charles Rice, "Report of the Committee on the Revision of the U.S. Pharmacopoeia," *Proc. Amer. Pharm. Ass.* 26 (1878): 670.
35. "Department of Graduate Study," in University of Wisconsin, *Catalogue*, 1895–96, p. 46.
36. *Proc. Amer. Pharm. Ass.* 45 (1897): 269.
37. David L. Cowen, "Louisiana, Pioneer in the Regulation of Pharmacy," *Louisiana Hist. Quart.* 26 (1943): 334–35.

century.[38] The legal control of drug adulteration varied, but commonly approximated section 16 of the model bill circulated in 1869, which made it a misdemeanor to:

> . . . knowlingly, intentionally and fraudulently adulterate or cause to be mixed any foreign or inert substance with any drug or medical substance, or any compound medicinal preparation recognized by the pharmacopoeia of the United States or of other countries as employed in medical practice, with the effect of weakening or destroying its medicinal power.[39]

This had the weaknesses of some of the earlier statutes, and the *Pharmacopoeia of the United States* is not given any status or force beyond that accorded to pharmacopoeias of other countries.

The proviso dealing with drug adulteration was omitted altogether from a revised model pharmacy act which the American Pharmaceutical Association issued at the turn of the century.[40] Instead of loss of interest, this reflected a transition toward separate and more comprehensive state laws on the subject.[41]

In a more limited sense, but on a broader base, the control of drug quality was reinforced by the general adoption of state laws during the closing decades of the century which legally defined the American pharmacist and his professional responsibilities. One responsibility, often stated explicitly, made the pharmacist guarantor of the quality of medicines he dispensed.[42] By the end of the century, however, the increasingly complex methods for checking the quality specifications of many drugs were becoming impracticable for even the best-equipped prescription laboratories in the country. Under the first federal Food and Drug Law (1906) the legal responsibility for drug quality was shifted from the practicing pharmacist to his suppliers, if they had offered a guaranty and if the product was dispensed as prefabricated, unchanged.[43]

38. Sonnedecker, *Kremers and Urdang's History of Pharmacy*, pp. 196–97.

39. *Proc. Amer. Pharm. Ass.* 56 (1869): 746.

40. James H. Beal, "A General Form of Pharmacy Law Suitable for Enactment by the Several States of the United States," *Proc. Amer. Pharm. Ass.* 48 (1900): 309–18.

41. It may have been a factor in the shift that "to carry on such work [against adulteration] systematically and continuously requires such expenditures as have never been granted to any state pharmacy board" under the statutes. Editorial, *Bull Amer. Pharm. Ass.* 5 (1910): 391.

42. See *Proc. Amer. Pharm. Ass.* 30 (1882): 487 (Iowa), 495 (W. Va.), 501 (Wis.); 39 (1891): 166 (Ore.), 167 (Wash.). Usually excepted were drugs in unbroken packages prefabricated by others.

43. While pharmacists were deeply divided about this expansion of governmental power, the *Pharmaceutical Era* editorialized that "state regulation has been fairly tried, and the discovery made that State lines have little force in maintaining standards for food and drugs . . . ." *Pharm. Era* 14 (1895): 512. The nineteenth-century statutes disappeared in most states, which soon modeled their intrastate regulation upon the pattern of the federal interstate authority. "Report of the Committee on Drug Reform," *Bull. Amer. Pharm. Ass.* 5 (1910): 655.

Role of Specifications. Although in 1900 it remained an unsettled issue whether the federal government should, or could, like that in many other countries, define and enforce specifications for drugs, a number of state laws had by then made reference to the U. S. *Pharmacopoeia.* In 1881, for example, New Jersey termed a drug adulterated "If, when sold under or by a name recognized in the United States Pharmacopoeia, it differs from the standard of strength, quality, or purity laid down therein" or from "the professed standard under which it is sold." The following year a Louisiana statute utilized pharmacopoeial standards in a similar way.[44]

Even in the absence of legal sanction, the *Pharmacopoeia* grew in authority among practitioners of the health professions, who increasingly referred to its standards as "official." Thus it exemplified the initiative and democratic action through voluntary association that are so embedded in the American tradition.

This associative endeavor relied increasingly upon pharmaceutical cooperation and interest after the 1860's. Several circumstances help account for this change. First, and perhaps most important, drafting specifications for drugs had become an increasingly complex scientific task, for which the knowledge of pharmacists with advanced training was more serviceable than that of physicians. Second, for pharmacists the *Pharmacopoeia* came to seem a bulwark against pre-emption of their traditional role by ready-made drugs with fanciful trade names and often with secret compositions, while for physicians the *Pharmacopoeia* may have seemed even less an indispensable guide to prescribing after the emergence of an important class of proprietary specialties. Moreover, a pharmacist whose living depended upon his knowledge of drugs, and upon his reputation for providing unwavering quality in pharmaceutical service, could best appreciate the significance of reliable and impartial standards. Third, the American Pharmaceutical Association took greater initiative in pharmacopoeial affairs after the late 1870's, perhaps partly motivated by a feeling that the two aging physicians who had borne the brunt of pharmacopoeial work from the first revision through the fifth were not fully adequate, scientifically or administratively, to new needs.[45]

In 1880 a special committee of the Association proposed not only a new edition but also a new type of pharmacopoeia.[46] The Chairman of this

---

44. "Report on Legislation," *Proc. Amer. Pharm. Ass.* 29 (1881): 394; S. Wolff, *Louisiana Constitution and Revised Laws of Louisiana,* 2d ed., vol. 2, p. 1469. Cf. Pennsylvania P. L. 85 of 1897, through *Purdon's Digest,* vol. 1, p. 326.

45. *Amer. J. Pharm.* 49 (1877): 518.

46. Charles Rice, *Report on the Revision of the U.S. Pharmacopoeia, Preliminary to the Convention of 1880* (New York: American Pharmaceutical Association, 1880). Voluntary contributions from pharmacists and organizations of pharmacy funded the printing and distribution of 2,000 copies nationally for criticism and suggestions. *Proc. Amer. Pharm. Ass.* 28 (1880): 528.

Committee, Charles Rice of New York, was elected Chairman of the Committee of Revision and Publication of the *Pharmacopoeia* itself. He was the first pharmacist to head the work, and for the first time a majority of the posts on the Committee were given to pharmacists.[47] Based upon the American Pharmaceutical Association report, the *Pharmacopoeia* of 1882 thus reflected a far-reaching reform led by pharmacists.[48]

The increased number of tests for identity and purity and the more meaningful description of physical and chemical characteristics of pharmacopoeial drugs implied that the focal point for producing and testing drugs was moving away from the local pharmacy. Yet the contents of the *Pharmacopoeia* remained core knowledge for every graduate pharmacist, and state regulations reflected an assumption that it should be in every pharmacy. Thus it has been primarily the pharmacists who have underwritten the cost of the pharmacopoeial program through purchase of the book, as later they underwrote a companion volume, the *National Formulary*.

Unlike the *Pharmacopoeia*, the *National Formulary of Unofficinal Preparations* (first edition, 1888) from the beginning has been prepared principally by pharmacists and published under the authority of their national professional society. Although the title of the first edition made explicit its "unofficinal" status, a few state laws recognized the *National Formulary* by 1900, and the others followed after the federal act of 1906 gave the *National Formulary* and *United States Pharmacopoeia* equal recognition. The phrase "of Unofficinal Preparations" disappeared from the title page of subsequent editions.[49]

The original purpose of the *National Formulary* was to provide standard formulae for the large number of nonproprietary preparations prescribed by physicians or demanded by the public which were not recognized by the *Pharmacopoeia*, and to relieve pharmacists of the necessity of stocking a variety of brands of what was nominally the same preparation.[50] In the second edition (1896), the American Pharmaceutical Association enunciated an objective that has been central ever since: to provide

47. For biographical information, see H. G. Wolfe, "Charles Rice (1841–1901), an Immigrant in Pharmacy," *Amer. J. Pharm. Educ.* 14 (1950): 285–305; England, *The First Century*, pp. 407–8.

48. George Urdang, "The Rescue of the United States Pharmacopoeia by Organized American Pharmacy in the 1870s," *Amer. J. Pharm. Educ.* 15 (1951): 172–84.

49. Concerning the transition, see G. Sonnedecker and G. Urdang, "Legalization of Drug Standards Under State Laws," *Food Drug Cosmet. Law J.* 8 (1953): 749–50, 753–54.

50. *The National Formulary of Unofficinal Preparations* (n.p.: American Pharmaceutical Association, 1888), p. iii. This resumed in modified form an interest of the Association expressed already in the 1860's by an earlier Committee on Unofficinal Formulas. *Proc. Amer. Pharm. Ass.* 18 (1870): 63. "A Preliminary Draft of a National Formulary of Unofficinal Preparations" appeared in *ibid.* 34 (1886): 191–285, and also as a separate.

standards for drugs omitted from the *Pharmacopoeia* and to serve as a proving ground for drugs that might be transferred to the *Pharmacopoeia* later.

At first the pharmacists working on the *National Formulary* contributed to controlling the quality of drugs mainly by standardizing the nomenclature and composition of medications identified as "N.F." Soon after 1900 the changing status of the *National Formulary* stimulated the elaboration of its drug specifications to a scientific level analogous with those of the *United States Pharmacopoeia*. This mutuality of endeavor without duplication of function produced an enduring collaboration between the two drug standardizing bodies that has earned international respect for America's "official" program of drug standardization.

Summary

This review of the contribution of the pharmaceutical profession toward controlling the quality of drugs in the nineteenth century suggests the following central trends:

1. Three changes merit first mention: (*a*) By the end of the century a legally defined, responsible group, moving in directions characteristic of a profession, had emerged, where none existed in 1800. (*b*) The very word "control" seems almost anomalous within the American context for three-quarters of the nineteenth century, even in a field so directly related to health. (*c*) The term "quality," at the century's beginning, implied little more than organoleptic sensing of basic ingredients and artful adherence to correct formula and procedure in preparing a medication; in 1900 the term "quality" comprised a complex of qualitative and quantitative descriptions, tests, and analyses.

2. While pharmacists have received increasing responsibility in the control of distribution, usage, and representation of the merits of drugs, they have felt a particular mission for control of quality.

3. There have always been knowledgeable American pharmacists who could be relied upon to give physician or patient as much assurance of drug quality as their resources permitted. However, during at least three-quarters of the nineteenth century, such men may have been a minority among the bulk of unorganized, uneducated, and uncontrolled drug dispensers.

4. The development of national systems of pharmaceutical organization and education and the legal definition of qualification and responsibility, mainly after the Civil War, magnified the meaningfulness of the pharmaceutical profession's contribution toward controlling the quality of drugs.

5. The control over the quality of drugs exercised by the average pharmacist, while meaningful and significant, has had an unfulfilled

potential. Just when organized efforts and educational preparation seemed to promise more, this function was undermined by changes in the technology and science of drug production and testing, and often by a commercial environment and underutilization of skills.

6. American confidence in the purifying effect of competition was eroded late in the century by influences such as the Populist movement, the exposure of substandard drugs by new scientific means, and a wider understanding (among both the health professions and educated laymen) of the difficulties in voluntary evaluation and control of quality variations in a highly technical field. As a consequence, organized pharmacists played a key role in bringing about the early legal controls: the federal act of 1848 controlling adulteration of drug imports, and the state pharmacy acts relating to licensing and adulteration.

7. An organized and consequential minority of pharmacists initiated early efforts to control drug quality and drug adulterators (at least in particular regions and periods) through such measures as sampling and checking the quality of drugs on the market, ethical sanctions against drug adulteration, experimental work to devise drug specifications and tests, and publication of literature to create information and attitudes fostering the control of drug quality.

8. Pharmacists contributed increasingly, from the 1830's onward, to enhancing the scientific quality and practical authority of the *United States Pharmacopoeia*, and near the end of the century they created a companion volume, the *National Formulary*, which reinforced the *Pharmacopoeia* as a medium for defining and controlling the quality of drugs.

From the intertwining of American developments and European patterns a distinctively American system of drug control emerged at the end of the nineteenth century, the principal outlines of which still can be perceived today. The pharmacist's acceptance of his role in this system was implicit in William Procter, Jr.'s statement of the pharmacist's duties: "*To procure and keep good drugs—to prepare from these, efficient and uniform medicines—to dispense these medicines to the sick in a perfect condition.*"[51]

51. William Procter, Jr., *Valedictory Charge to the Graduates of the Philadelphia College of Pharmacy, delivered . . . 1855* (Philadelphia: Kite and Walton, 1855), p. 9.

The Prescription-Drug Policies
of the American Medical Association
in the Progressive Era

James G. Burrow

Problems that seemed more urgent than drug issues confronted the American Medical Association just as the twentieth century began. The struggling organization, numbering only 8,400 physicians, or less than one-twelfth of the regular medical profession, could not overcome the sluggishness of half a century or the divisive forces of the healing world with concern for purely scientific matters. Its leadership assigned priority to the task of remodeling the profession's archaic organizational structure and transforming a largely sectional society into a strong and thriving national organization. Only when this work got under way could it deal seriously with some of the most important scientific matters.

The AMA saw formidable obstructions to the advance of scientific medicine in the early twentieth century. Prosperous proprietary establishments multiplied in an environment that had long cultivated what Professor James Harvey Young has called "medical democracy."[1] The contradictory claims of sectarian medicine persisted; there were inadequate means for assessing their validity. Peripheral religious and occult groups emphasizing spiritual and psychic healing often threatened the progress of scientific medicine. The remarkable advance of preventive medicine raised untimely doubts about even the survival of any therapeutic system. Within the regular profession itself, despair and defeatism over the retarded development of drug therapy perpetuated a spirit of therapeutic nihilism. In 1903 Frank Billings, the President of the AMA, expressed what probably a large part of the profession believed when he told the House of Delegates that with the exception of quinine for malaria and mercury for syphilis drugs were "valueless as cures." Five years later Torald Sollmann of the AMA's Council on Pharmacy and Chemistry wrote that therapeutics could be considered as neither an art nor a science but only confusion. Yet he held out hope, adding that "the present turbidity . . . is the turbidity of fermentation, rather than that of putre-faction."[2]

1. James Harvey Young, "American Medical Quakery in the Age of the Common Man," *Mississippi Valley Hist. Rev.* 47 (March, 1961): 592.
2. Frank Billings, "Medical Education in the United States," *JAMA* 40 (May 9, 1903): 1273; Torald Sollmann, "The Broader Aims of the Council on Pharmacy and Chemistry," *JAMA* 50 (April 4, 1908): 1134.

However much therapeutic nihilism may have flourished within the profession, it should not obscure the AMA's effort to institute measures of drug reform in the Progressive Era. In the first issue of the *Journal of the American Medical Association* in the twentieth century, the new editor, George H. Simmons, applauded an appeal of the Secretary of Agriculture urging a congressional appropriation for an investigation of medicinal flora in the United States and for experimentation with the culture of nonindigenous medicinal plants. The following year, President Charles A. L. Reed lamented that the request had been denied even a "courteous consideration" and reminded the St. Paul session that the Association's own investigation, begun more than four decades earlier, had never been completed.[3]

The Association made no effort to resume a botanical investigation, but gradually turned to more realistic tasks. Although it had shown no interest in the pharmacopoeial revision in 1900, it joined with the American Pharmaceutical Association about two years later in establishing a committee to study such problems as drug efficacy and adulteration. After careful consideration this committee proposed a "National Bureau of Medicines and Foods" which would certify the "identity, purity, quality and strength" of the pharmaceutical preparations that it accepted.[4]

The committee acknowledged that the functions assigned to this bureau properly belonged to an agency of the federal government, but added that all efforts to secure federal control had failed. This bureau, to be financed by manufacturers accepting its services, would make reports on its drug investigations available to pharmacists and physicians. Although the proposal divorced the AMA from any financial responsibility or legal liability, for undisclosed reasons the House of Delegates in June, 1904, rejected the Committee's request. The delegates also failed to act on a resolution proposing a "Journal Clearing House Commission" with authority to have analyses made by reliable laboratories or to establish a suitable laboratory for that purpose.[5]

When the House of Delegates appeared to offer no direction, the persistent group urging drug investigation upon the AMA revised its strategy. It decided not only that the Association should act alone in establishing a drug investigating agency but also, apparently, that a body reporting directly to the Board of Trustees could be created solely by the Board. In contrast to the Association's years of indecision the Board approved the establishment of the Council on Pharmacy and

3. *JAMA* 34 (January 6, 1900): 49, 50; *JAMA* 35 (June 8, 1901): 1601.
4. M. G. Motter, *JAMA* 51 (December 12, 1908): 2027; *JAMA* 40 (June 20, 1903): 1736–37.
5. *JAMA* 42 (June 18, 1904): 1640, 1644; George H. Simmons, "The Commercial Domination of Therapeutics and the Movement for Reform," *JAMA* 48 (May 18, 1907): 1646.

Chemistry only days before the newly created body held its first meeting in Pittsburgh on February 11, 1905.[6]

For several reasons the establishment of the Council marks an important event in the Association's history. Through the Council the AMA for the first time moved with considerable effectiveness against forces resisting the slow advance of rational therapy. For the first time it made a serious effort to restore professional confidence in ethical drugs and therapeutics. It also represented the Association's attempt to appropriate the new techniques of drug analysis for a very important public and professional use. Finally, it indicated the AMA's effort to gain a measure of disciplinary power over the drug industry that would perhaps be more effective than it could have expected of any governmental regulation.[7]

At first the Council confined its investigations to ethical proprietaries, only later broadening its work to include analyses of preparations sold directly to the public. It issued an annual publication, *New and Nonofficial Remedies*, to inform the profession of products conforming to the ten rules of admission. The Council's acceptance required full revelation of all medicinal ingredients and their amount in any given quantity of an article and submission of information regarding tests for determining its identity, purity, and strength. It insisted that, when an article bore an insufficiently descriptive trade name, it should have another name indicating its "chemical composition or pharmaceutical character." It accepted almost no articles advertised to the public and none that carried false or exaggerated claims. Later it amended a rule to specify rejection of "useless" preparations, though it insisted from the beginning that it had power only to accept or reject, not to approve, any product.[8]

No brief treatment can adequately indicate the scope and effectiveness of the Council's work, but both could be measured by the cries of its critics. Just as the Council included acceptable preparations in *New and Nonofficial Remedies*, it soon raised the wrath of many manufacturers by exposing rejected articles in the Association's *Journal*. One of its members listed the cardinal faults of proprietaries as intentional deception, secrecy as to composition, and exploitation to the public, but added that more had been rejected for having been surreptitiously advertised to the

6. *JAMA* 48 (May 18, 1907): 1646; "Report of Board of Trustees," *JAMA* 52 (June 19, 1909): 2034.
7. For late nineteenth-century progress in the analysis of drugs and the detection of adulteration, see Ernst W. Stieb, with the collaboration of Glenn Sonnedecker, *Drug Adulteration: Detection and Control in Nineteenth-Century Britain* (Madison: University of Wisconsin Press, 1966), p. 203 and *passim*.
8. "Report of the Council on Pharmacy and Chemistry," *JAMA* 45 (July 22, 1905): 265; W. A. Puckner, "The Council on Pharmacy and Chemistry, Present and Future," in *The Propaganda for Reform in Proprietary Medicines*, vol. 2 (Chicago: American Medical Association, 1922), pp. 13–14; Sollmann, "Broader Aims of the Council," *JAMA* 50 (May 9, 1908): 1540.

public than for all other causes combined. In July, 1907, George H. Simmons wrote that the new agency had already considered 600 preparations and had approved nearly 300. The Council did not confine its inspection to products voluntarily submitted but watched the medical journals for articles advertised with suspicious claims. So great did the Council's work become that the AMA established its own Chemical Laboratory in the fall of 1906.[9]

When it established the Council, the Association had held only a faint hope that the federal government would move as soon as it did against drug abuses. It had underestimated the impact of its own agitation and that of allied groups struggling for reform. Nor could it foresee the national shock brought on by the publication of Upton Sinclair's book *The Jungle*, a year to the month after the creation of the Council, or the feeling stirred by Samuel Hopkins Adams' articles on medical quackery, which completed their run in *Collier's* during the same month that *The Jungle* appeared. The Pure Food and Drugs Act passed five months later formally allied the federal government with the AMA in a struggle to destroy the nostrum menace and to protect the public against adulterated drugs. The law established the *United States Pharmacopoeia* and the *National Formulary* as standards of strength and purity for drugs, and, whatever its inadequacies, the AMA welcomed the measure as a distinct advance.[10]

The passage of the new legislation strengthened the Association's effort to promote the purity and efficacy of prescription drugs but did not blind the AMA to the law's deficiencies. Less than six months after the legislation became effective, a Council member, Carl S. N. Hallberg, warned the profession of some of these inadequacies. The law, he observed, did not require all articles of the *Pharmacopoeia* and the *National Formulary* to conform to these standards if the label specifically indicated a different strength and quality. Tincture of opium with an official strength of 10 per cent might be manufactured at 5 per cent, and morphine with an official strength of 1.2 per cent might be only 1 per cent. He charged that chemicals had already been sold that fell below the official requirements as to quality, purity, and strength.

Hallberg also criticized the law for applying the labeling restrictions regarding the presence of alcohol and some of the habit-forming drugs to physicians' prescriptions and to articles of the *Pharmacopoeia* and the *National Formulary*. Prescriptions, he said, seldom entered interstate commerce, and standards for the other items were already set. Furthermore,

9. *JAMA* 50 (May 9, 1908): 1541; *JAMA* 50 (April 18, 1908): 1280; letter, George H. Simmons to Philip Mills Jones, July 9, 1907, in *J. Kansas Med. Soc.* 7 (November 1, 1907): 1141.

10. James G. Burrow, *AMA: Voice of American Medicine* (Baltimore: Johns Hopkins Press, 1963), pp. 77–83; James Harvey Young, *The Toadstool Millionaires* (Princeton: Princeton University Press, 1961), pp. 217–23; 34 U.S. *Statutes* 768.

he warned that manufacturers often sold chemicals like magnesium carbonate in large packages labeled "for technical purposes," but that the law required no label on smaller quantities sold from the package to retail pharmacists. Frequently these chemicals contained such poisonous substances as heavy-metal salts, which pharmacists could easily dispense unknowingly.[11]

As the AMA was revealing defects in the federal law, it did not overlook the problem of drug regulation within the states. Most states had enacted food and drug laws before 1906, but they were weak and inadequately enforced. Hallberg urged the AMA to seek removal from state legislation of the objectionable features appearing in the national law, such as the inclusion of physicians' prescriptions in the regulations on alcohol and the habit-forming drugs, and allowance for deviation from the standards of the *Pharmacopoeia* and the *National Formulary* if the label of a preparation revealed its actual quality.[12]

The AMA upheld the revised laws of Kentucky and Tennessee as the most satisfactory and publicized these statutes in pamphlet form. It urged the profession to seek similar legislation in all states.[13] The Kentucky law of March 13, 1908, defined an adulterated article as one whose "strength or purity fall[s] below the professed standard under which it is sold" or one in which "a greater or less quantity of any ingredient specified . . . is used than that prescribed." Adulterated articles also normally included those sold under names recognized in the *Pharmacopoeia* and the *National Formulary* but differing from the official standards in "strength, quality and purity." Although the law excluded physicians' prescriptions from the regulations governing alcohol and habit-forming drugs, it incorporated the variations clause of the national legislation so sharply criticized by Hallberg, allowing deviations from the standards of the *Pharmacopoeia* and the *National Formulary* when the label of an article stated its standard of "strength, quality and purity." The Kentucky law made generous concessions in administrative matters to the state medical and pharmaceutical associations. It authorized each of these bodies to select a representative every year to work with the director of the state experiment station in establishing "all rules and regulations" for administering the Act.[14]

11. C. S. N. Hallberg, "Pharmacists and Physicians and the Food and Drugs Act," *JAMA* 49 (October 26, 1907): 1413–14.
12. *JAMA* 49 (October 26, 1907): 1413; *JAMA* 56 (April 22, 1911): 1212; David Livingstone Dykstra, "Patent and Proprietary Medicines: Regulation Control Prior to 1906" (Ph.D. dissertation, University of Wisconsin, 1951), p. 106.
13. "Report of Committee on Medical Legislation," *JAMA* 50 (May 23, 1908): 1741; *JAMA* 50 (March 21, 1908): 985–86; *JAMA* 48 (May 18, 1907): 1692–93.
14. *JAMA* 48 (May 18, 1907): 1692–93; *Carroll's Kentucky Statutes*, 1909, Ch. 53a, par. 1905a.

The Association's advocacy of what it considered to be the most advanced state legislation soon gave way to a slightly different but abortive strategy. When, in April, 1908, the Twelfth Annual Convention of the State and National Food and Dairy Departments appointed a committee to draft a model pure food bill, the AMA quickly saw the possibility of enlarging the measure to include a drug section and of securing allies in the struggle for adoption. R. M. Allen, who had drafted the Kentucky law, presented the model food bill to the annual conference of the AMA's Committee on Medical Legislation in February, 1909. The Committee proposed to add a drug section to this measure and to urge its adoption throughout the nation. Very quickly, though, threatening legislative proposals in many state capitals diverted the Association from its purpose. It called upon the profession to repel the attacks of irregular healing groups seeking recognition and attempting to upset the licensing laws of many states. The model bill was a casualty in the struggle.[15]

Yet the Association recognized the limits of legislation in bringing drug reform. It knew that the most vigorous enforcement of drug statutes could not drive advertisements of many worthless proprietaries from the pages of even medical journals. Nor could legal recognition of the *Pharmacopoeia* and the *National Formulary* add to the scientific value of these standards. It knew that no drug measure could enhance in any way the physicians' qualifications to prescribe, and that professional training in materia medica and pharmacy had largely been deficient. In the years 1905–9 the AMA became painfully aware that the effectiveness of its struggle against adulterated and worthless ethical drugs depended not only upon its effort to improve and enforce drug legislation and to maintain its own machinery of investigation but also upon educating much of the profession in a scientific approach to drug therapy.

In attempting to drive worthless prescription drugs from the therapeutic field through a program of professional education, the American Medical Association soon realized the magnitude of its task. In June, 1907, a medical professor, M. Clayton Thrush, told the AMA's Section on Pharmacology and Therapeutics that not half of the profession had ever seen a copy of the *Pharmacopoeia*, not one-third had ever seen an issue of the *National Formulary*, and not one-tenth were ordering the new official preparations of the latest *Pharmacopoeia*. His careful investigation of the instruction offered by American medical colleges in pharmacy and materia medica revealed a range of from 15 to 300 hours in lectures

15. *JAMA* 51 (September 5, 1908): 858–59; "Report of Committee on Medical Legislation," *JAMA* 52 (June 19, 1909): 2042–43; "Report of Council on Health and Public Instruction," *JAMA* 57 (July 1, 1911): 64. The dominance of licensing issues over state food and drugs legislation is clearly indicated in the publications of the state medical associations early in the second decade.

and recitations, with one leading medical school covering the subjects of pharmacy, materia medica, and prescription writing in 15 classroom hours. A year later another educator lamented the profession's neglect of therapeutics and the fact that the Section on Pharmacology and Therapeutics remained the smallest in the Association.[16]

To Torald Sollmann, a member of the Council on Pharmacy and Chemistry, fell much of the task of instructing the profession in proper drug therapy. The *Journal* not only published several of his special articles but also one that appeared in twenty-two installments beginning in the issue of March 28, 1908. While condemning all forms of secret proprietary and nostrum therapy, he also emphasized the caution with which the *Pharmacopoeia* and the *National Formulary* should be used. In a special article he showed that although the Pure Food and Drugs Act had made these publications federal standards, the former was revised only once in a decade and always remained behind medical advances. It did not contain many useful remedies and included some that were obsolete. He described the *Formulary* as a "modest, unobtrusive, harmless and really useful little book" in which "the tottering great-grandmothers of the materia medica were resurrected from their therapeutic graveyard, to join in a merry dance with the lusty and vociferous youngsters of the modern therapeutic yellow press . . . ." To Sollmann, this publication of the American Pharmaceutical Association adhered closely to the idea that "For those who like this sort of thing, this is the sort of thing they like."[17] Its elevation to the position of a scientific standard had not enhanced its scientific value.

With equally penetrating articles another influential writer, Solomon Solis-Cohen, joined Sollmann in carrying the problem of drug therapy far beyond the use of nostrums. Solis-Cohen insisted that the chief objection to any proprietary lay in the fact that it was ready-made and could "no more fit the pathologic conditions in every patient, than one coat can fit the curves of every back." In most instances proprietaries contained unnecessary ingredients, omitted essential ingredients, or provided an improper balance. But he added that the same charge could be made about mixture formulas of the *Pharmacopoeia* and the *National Formulary*. He insisted that the two standards should publish skeleton formulas indicating "an optional range of variations possible," leaving the exact dosage to the

16. M. Clayton Thrush, "A Plea for a More Thorough Course in Practical Pharmacy and Prescription Dispensing in Our Medical Schools," *JAMA* 50 (January 25, 1908): 255–56; L. E. Sayre, "Some Ways and Means to Overcome the Practice of Prescribing Ready-Made Remedies and Proprietaries," *J. Missouri Med. Ass.* 5 (January, 1909): 425. Thrush's figures are taken from the catalogues of sixty-eight medical schools that showed the hours of instruction.
17. Torald Sollmann, "The Pharmacopoeia as the Standard for Medical Prescribing," *JAMA* 51 (December 12, 1908): 2017.

physician's judgment. As an example, he suggested that the *Pharmacopoeia* should indicate the range in which the preparations of tincture of chloride of iron and the solution of ammonium acetate should be varied in Basham's mixture.[18]

The AMA did not confine its educational crusade during the first decade to the pages of the *Journal*. It also attempted to sustain the interest of the local societies so recently established or revived with a "postgraduate course of study" that gave some attention to drugs and their action. In fact, physicians responding to an appeal for suggestions on the organization of the course expressed greatest interest in materia medica and therapeutics. In the fall of 1907 the AMA published the first six-month schedule, which John H. Blackburn of Bowling Green, Kentucky had so carefully prepared. As instruction to societies offering the course, Blackburn urged: "Study materia medica, pharmacology and therapeutics, exhibiting crude drugs and their U.S.P. and N.F. preparations. Encourage members or classes to carry out experiments on animals in regard to the effects of drugs." In June, 1909, he reported to the House of Delegates that 200 societies had begun the course and that interest had steadily increased.[19]

When the *Pharmacopoeia* and the *National Formulary* together contained 1,395 drugs and preparations, the AMA well knew that the profession needed something more than extensive pharmacological instruction to make its way through the confusion. Before the end of the decade it had issued not only several editions of *New and Nonofficial Remedies* but also a booklet entitled the *Epitome of the U.S. Pharmacopoeia and National Formulary*. This manual, which the Association sold for fifty cents, offered a systematic and convenient classification of drugs appearing in the two standards.[20] In addition, the AMA continued to offer assistance in guiding the profession around the pitfalls of prescription with the *Journal*'s exposure of many fraudulent proprietaries.

The AMA developed its machinery and most of its policies of drug reform in five years' time. In the period 1905–9, it appeared before the public and profession alike largely in an iconoclastic role. Its fierce attacks on the nostrum forces overshadow edits quieter effort to instruct and inspire the profession. In the second decade the organization lost neither this role nor this image, but its work entered a broader phase.

18. Solomon Solis-Cohen, "The Prescribing of Proprietaries, Especially Proprietary Mixtures," *JAMA* 51 (September 19, 1908): 989–90.
19. *JAMA* 50 (May 23, 1908): 1750; *JAMA* 52 (June 19, 1909): 2077; quotation, AMA *Councilor's Bull.* 3 (September 15, 1907): 9.
20. M. Clayton Thrush, "The U.S. Pharmacopoeia and the National Formulary," *JAMA* 54 (February 5, 1910): 436; Puckner, "The Council on Pharmacy and Chemistry," p. 14.

The Association's contribution to the pharmacopoeial revision of 1910 sharply contrasted with its virtual indifference in 1900. It also worked with schools of pharmacy and pharmaceutical organizations in such a way as to avoid reviving dying enmities. It made no effort to capture the *Pharmacopoeia*, as one prominent physician had proposed, but seems to have exercised considerable influence over the articles accepted or excluded in the revised compendium.[21]

In preparing for the revision, the AMA brought much of the strength of the organization into play. A special committee worked closely with the appointees of medical schools, who constituted 75 per cent of the medical delegates sent to the convention. It also secured the appointment of committees within the AMA's sections which circularized their membership for advice on drugs that should be included or excluded from the *Pharmacopoeia*. The committee of the Section of Ophthalmology, for example, after circularizing 930 members, recommended that six additional drugs useful in ophthalmology be added to the *Pharmacopoeia*. The special committee reported from its correspondence with delegates of medical schools that a majority recommended the deletion of 279 articles.[22]

As the AMA assumed greater responsibility for the *Pharmacopoeia*, it also sought stronger and more effective enforcement of federal drug legislation. Just as the new decade opened, it regained hope for the early establishment of a national health department and moved quickly to support the first Owen Bill. This Bill called for the creation of a bureau of food and drugs within the proposed health department and for the concentration within the bureau of all scattered governmental activities related to food and drugs. In supporting the measure Charles A. L. Reed, a spokesman for the AMA, urged that the bureau be empowered to establish standards for the purity of drugs and to conduct an extensive survey of medicinal flora in the United States. Despite persistent effort the Association failed in its agitation for a national health department, though it was partially gratified in 1912 when, through passage of the Sherley Amendment to the Pure Food and Drugs Act, the government secured greater control over proprietary advertising.[23]

Opposition aroused by the Owen Bill and later revisions convinced the AMA that the force of its campaign against the manufacturer of

21. Henry Leffmann, "What Physicians Can Do to Improve the Pharmacopoeia," *JAMA* 54 (February 5, 1910): 431–32; see also *ibid.*, p. 432, for remarks of Henry Beates of Philadelphia.

22. "Report of Committee of Section on Ophthalmology," *JAMA* 53 (September 4, 1909): 793–94; "Report of Committee on United States Pharmacopeia," *JAMA* 54 (June 18, 1910): 2088–90.

23. Letter, Reed to Robert Owen, March 10, 1910, *JAMA* 54 (March 19, 1910): 986; Burrow, *AMA*, pp. 90–91, 96–104; James Harvey Young, *The Medical Messiahs: A Social History of Health Quackery in Twentieth-Century America* (Princeton: Princeton University Press, 1967), pp. 49–51.

worthless and harmful proprietaries must not diminish. Although the *Journal* had long exposed objectionable proprietaries sold to both the profession and the public, it had never collected these exposures in book form. In 1911 it published the first volume of *Nostrums and Quackery*, which concentrated on proprietaries sold to the public, and about the same time it struck at worthless proprietaries advertised to physicians, in the first volume of *The Propaganda for Reform in Proprietary Medicines*. The favorable reception given these volumes quickly assured the AMA of the wisdom of this publishing venture.[24]

Just as the Association put physicians on guard against objectionable proprietaries with these two books, it published another volume about two years later to reduce the bewilderment of the *Pharmacopoeia*. This book, entitled *Useful Drugs*, included articles of the *Pharmacopoeia* that the Association considered most valuable. It found immediate use in several medical schools, which adopted it as a text, and by at least one medical examining board, which accepted it as an examination guide.[25]

The AMA's struggle to promote the efficacy of prescription drugs also took a more constructive turn in the second decade of the twentieth century. Understandably, some of the dying sectarian medical groups resented the Association's attacks on their therapeutic systems when the organization itself had failed to contribute significantly to drug research. In 1908 a committee of the American Institute of Homoeopathy unsuccessfully challenged the Association to participate in a joint scientific investigation of the merits of the homeopathic system of drug selection, and three years later an Eclectic editor attacked the Council on Pharmacy and Chemistry for consistently belittling "the therapeutic action of the kindly plant remedies."[26] In 1912 the AMA established the Committee on Therapeutic Research, which began to foster investigations of "the activity, stability and physiologic action of commonly used nonproprietary drugs," and within a year had appropriated $3,500 for its studies. In 1915 the Board of Trustees announced that the Committee's work would restore to their proper places well-known drugs that had been sacrificed by commercial proprietary propaganda. Within less than a decade the Committee had conducted investigations that included "the action of strychnin in cardiac disease," the "pharmacology of the opium alkaloids," and "a comparison of the actions of absorption and excretion of iodid preparations."[27]

24. Burrow, *AMA*, pp. 110–11.
25. "Report of Board of Trustees," *JAMA* 60 (June 21, 1913): 1989; *JAMA* 63 (July 4, 1914): 75.
26. *J. Amer. Inst. Homoeop.* 5 (June, 1913): 1352–53; *Eclectic Med. J.* 71 (April, 1911): 206.
27. "Special Report of the Work of the Council on Pharmacy and Chemistry," *JAMA* 65 (July 3, 1915): 69–70; Puckner, "The Council on Pharmacy and Chemistry," p. 15.

Nearly two years before the entrance of the United States into World War I closed the Progressive Era, the AMA reflected on the drug struggles of a decade. The Council on Pharmacy and Chemistry claimed important victories. It had battled with considerable effectiveness against the manufacturers of worthless proprietaries which had deceived and misguided the profession. As the complexities of scientific medicine had increased, so also had its own effort to instruct the profession, with some measure of success. Its attempt to encourage the teaching of pharmacology in medical schools as a part of the AMA's program of educational reform had been unusually rewarding.

Nevertheless, the Council gave greater attention to the darker side. It bitterly criticized the profession for still tolerating "so-called 'ethical proprietaries'" that were "as fraudulent as many of the 'patent medicines' . . . ." It complained that a large part of the medical press remained subservient to proprietary interests and hostile to its own work. The Council believed that drug research as then conducted offered little hope. It maintained that the medical profession had never discovered more than "a score or so of the really useful drugs" and that commercialism had dominated and largely ruined the research activities of private firms. Citing the retarded state of American drug research, it concluded: "It is only from laboratories free from any relation with manufacturers that real advances can be expected."[28]

The AMA set goals in the Progressive Era that were far beyond its reach. The necessity of political combat on many fronts, and the weakness of its own political organization, partially prevented greater success in securing more effective drug legislation. As a result of the meager training of a large part of the profession, the AMA's insistence on a scientific approach to drug therapy could have been only moderately successful. Nor could it settle questions about the efficacy of drugs that even now remain obscure. It was in no financial position to encourage extensive drug research, nor could it have secured adequate funds from other sources. Its crusade against the advertising of worthless proprietaries could not wholly succeed among medical publications struggling desperately for survival.

Actually, the AMA was near the dawn of a brighter era. Its own Council and Chemical Laboratory were to regulate the manufacture of American synthetic drugs after the United States entered the war, and within a few years there would be major breakthroughs in drug research. By insisting on an approach that encouraged scientific research and experimentation and by sweeping away many obstructions to medical advance, the AMA contributed to the triumphs of later decades.

28. "Special Report of the Work of the Council," *JAMA* 65 (July 3, 1915): 69 and 69n.

The American Medical Association's Policy on Drugs in Recent Decades

Harry F. Dowling

Among the private agencies involved in the regulation of drugs, the American Medical Association has invested the largest amount of money and effort during the past sixty years. Its endeavors fall into three periods, which I have called anticipatory, regulatory, and educational. The first extended from the formation of the AMA in 1847 to the establishment of the Council on Pharmacy and Chemistry in 1905; the second, until 1955, when the Seal of Acceptance program was dropped; and the third, from 1955 to the present.

The Anticipatory and Regulatory Periods

The anticipatory period was marked by complaints from physicians that they could not tell what was in many of the widely advertised drugs and by criticisms of the AMA *Journal* for accepting questionable advertisements.

The regulatory era began with the formation of a strong Council on Pharmacy and Chemistry, which was effective because (1) some of the nation's top experts were on it; (2) the AMA staff was militantly behind its program; and (3) it early fashioned a club which it was to wield effectively for the next half-century, the Seal of Acceptance program. This meant that the *Journal* of the AMA and affiliated journals would not accept advertising for a drug unless the drug was fully identified and met standards of efficacy and toxicity set by the Council, and unless advertising for the drug was truthful. The editor of the *Journal* backed the Council policies with telling articles and vigorous speeches. By 1920 the Council could claim that the "complex mixtures of simple drugs exploited to our profession under fanciful names and with extravagant claims" had been forced into obscurity.[1]

During the regulatory period the AMA was continually watching over the advertising in its journals. The editor of the *Journal* was chairman of the Advertising Committee. The secretary of the Council examined all

1. "Report of the Board of Trustees," *JAMA* 76 (June 11, 1921): 1657–60.

This research was supported by PHS Grant No. 5 Fl3 LM 26,400 from the National Library of Medicine.

advertisements and either rejected them or advised rewriting if the claims were excessive. The Advertising Committee almost always accepted his decisions, but in the case of a disagreement, the final decision rested with the editor.

Gradually, the outright quacks and the fringe operators were forced out of the *Journal*'s advertising columns and sometimes out of business too. The leading companies swung around to a conformity which, though grudging, yet resulted in better quality products and more realistic statements about them. In 1910 the editor had complained that "two directly related interests—the so-called ethical proprietary business and the 'patent medicine' business—by fair means and foul have done their best to discredit and injure the Association."[2] In contrast, in 1946 the Board of Trustees could rejoice that "the Council's office has been swamped with presentations of products from firms who are now striving to bring their policies into conformance with Council principles . . . ."[3]

Revenue from advertising surpassed that from dues and journal subscriptions in 1919. It fell behind later, but between 1950 and 1954 it rose steadily from $2,500,000 to $3,250,000, although this was still less than other income, which remained at around $5,000,000.[4]

Then in 1955, in spite of the rising income from advertising, in spite of the continuous growth of the Council's program, in spite of statements of approval by the Board of Trustees, the Council suddenly dropped its Seal of Acceptance program. Why this was done will be examined more closely later; for the present let us look at the activities of the AMA during the following period.

The Educational Period

The personnel of the Council was changed by dropping the representatives from the federal government and the editor of the *JAMA* and adding practicing physicians. Membership on all councils of the AMA was limited to ten years and the chairmanship to three years. This meant that doctors who had been on the Council for many years were dropped, including its doughty chairman Torald Sollmann, author of the textbook of pharmacology that had nurtured a generation of physicians.

Whether as a result of changes in personnel and continuity or the loss of the Seal program, the Council steered a shifting course for the

2. "The American Medical Association—Its Policies and Its Work," *JAMA* 54 (March 5, 1910): 796–97.
3. "Proceedings of the Chicago Session . . . December 9–11, 1946," *JAMA* 132 (Dec. 21, 1946): 997.
4. U.S. Congress, Senate, Committee on the Judiciary, *Drug Industry Antitrust Act; Hearings before the Subcommittee on Antitrust and Monopoly . . . on S. 1552*, 87th Cong., 1st sess., July 5–25, 1961, pt. 1 (Washington: Government Printing Office, 1961), p. 129.

next few years. In 1955 it announced an "expanded program" for gathering, evaluating, and disseminating information about drugs. But this program was strongly dependent on the submission of data on new drugs by the pharmaceutical manufacturers, and many of them saw no reason to comply. The club was gone; the Council and the editor of the *Journal* no longer controlled its advertising columns.

Although the main thrust of the Council was now educational, the doctors did not read what the Council said! The annual publication was renamed *New Drugs* and modified to attract the practicing physician. This helped, but still only 31,000 copies were sold in the peak year, 1966.

Spurred by deaths from aplastic anemia in patients who had received chloramphenicol, Dr. Maxwell Wintrobe in 1953 formed a Committee on Blood Dyscrasias under the Council, which was later broadened to include all adverse reactions to drugs. This committee set up a registry so that physicians in private practice and in hospitals could report adverse reactions. The program resulted in a number of reports being sent to the Council which were used as the basis of several articles on adverse reactions to drugs.[5] But the program had deficiencies: only a fraction of all adverse reactions were reported; there was no way of knowing how many patients had received the drug which caused reactions in some; and, finally, all the reactions reported were already known. Nevertheless, the program was an important step toward more exact systems of reporting, which the Food and Drug Administration and the Public Health Service are just getting in motion today.

In one area the Council marched forward without breaking step. When the Seal program was in effect, the name of the drug was negotiated between the Council and the manufacturer and was used in all publications and advertisements in AMA journals. This gave the Council bargaining power, which it had lost when it dropped its Seal of Acceptance. To regain this power, the Council joined the U.S. Pharmacopeia in 1961 to form a Committee on Nomenclature. In 1964 this was broadened to include a representative of the *National Formulary* and named the United States Adopted Names (USAN) Council.

Since the Drug Amendments Act of 1962 gave the Secretary of Health, Education, and Welfare power to choose a generic name for a drug when he considered the one in use unsuitable, a representative of the FDA was added in 1967. The Commissioner of Food and Drugs agreed to accept any name adopted unanimously. If the Council's decision was

5. "Blood Dyscrasias Associated with Chlorpromazine Therapy," *JAMA* 160 (Jan. 28, 1956): 287; "Blood Dyscrasias Associated with Chloramphenicol (Chloromycetin) Therapy," *JAMA* 172 (April 30, 1960): 2044–45; C. M. Huguley, Jr., A. J. Erslev, and D. E. Bergsagel, "Drug-related Blood Dyscrasias," *JAMA* 177 (July 8, 1961): 23–26.

not unanimous, the Commissioner reserved the right to designate an official name.[6] Thus a regulatory program was begun by a private group, strengthened by the incorporation of other groups, and eventually given official status when the government joined it. The private groups, representing as they do the physicians, pharmacists, and the drug industry, still help to select names; yet the requirements of government as they reflect the interests of the public are served, without complete government controls.

Changes in Policy

Having considered the actions of the AMA with respect to drugs during the anticipatory, regulatory, and educational periods, let us look at the reasons for its shifts in policy, taking up first its abandonment of the Seal of Acceptance program. Senator Kefauver charged that the AMA had done this to sell more advertising. The AMA's witnesses gave other reasons: (1) the Seal program took up too much of the Council's time; (2) it was too arbitrary and vested too much authority in one body; and (3) there were "legal problems."

What can be said of these purported reasons? The volume of work required in evaluating new drugs is indeed tremendous, but this was hardly lessened by dropping the Seal program; in fact, the difficulties were increased because the drug companies no longer had a compelling reason to submit data to the AMA. Thus, much time of the staff is now spent in getting information from other sources.

The second claim, that the program vested too much authority in a small group, is one which will always be made by the regulated against the regulators. It is being made now against the Food and Drug Administration. While the Seal program was in effect, two groups were evaluating drugs, the AMA and the FDA; now there is only one. Thus the drug companies actually had more leeway under the old system.

Finally, the threat of civil suits should not have been overriding when we recall the barrage of suits against the AMA in the early 1900's from which the Association had emerged vindicated, honored, and applauded. A suit by the federal government for restraint of trade would have been more serious, but close liaison with the FDA and strict adherence to scientific evidence in rejecting drugs should have prevented this.

Why then was the program abandoned? For a private agency to regulate successfully, five forces are necessary: consecration, crusading, consistent pressure, clubs, and cash. One needs only to read the editorials in *JAMA* in the early decades of the century to be convinced that the consecration was there. And to follow the speeches and the actions of

6. "USAN, FDA Compromise: Agreement on Drug Names," *AMA News*, Aug. 21, 1967, p. 2.

Simmons and Fishbein, to watch how they braved criticism, vilification, and legal prosecution, is to see militant, courageous crusaders in action. But Simmons died, and Fishbein was dropped from the AMA staff and was not replaced by an equally militant champion, and eventually all staff members of the AMA were removed from the Council.

The third force, consistent pressure, was applied in the early years of the Council when a chairman such as Torald Sollmann remained at the helm and when the editor of the *Journal* attended every meeting, but this force was effectively braked when the term of membership in councils was limited and chairmen could serve for only three years.

Regulation seldom if ever succeeds by persuasion alone; some kind of a club is needed. The Seal of Acceptance was such a club. It helped to keep the large companies in line, while the smaller companies scrambled to be in the ranks with them. Perhaps the club was not big enough, because, after World War II, the drug companies had released a flood of drugs on the market—new compounds, duplicate compounds, and mixtures. Also the Madison Avenue methodologies had taken over drug advertising, and the pages of medical journals bulged with glowing testimonials. Yet a bigger club might have cost too much.

And that brings us to the final requirement. A regulatory program takes cash, and lots of it, and the lack of cash may be the real rock on which the Seal program foundered. In 1955 the AMA had just come through the searing experience of prosecution and conviction for criminal violation of the antitrust laws. The fine it had to pay was trivial, but the costs of the legal battle were not. Moreover, the AMA was mounting a costly campaign to prevent government payment for medical care, and the accusation by the government that the AMA was restraining trade might well have been echoed by some drug company whose products were not approved; this would have cost more money! Added to these factors was the glimpse of a treasure chest of potential advertising from which the AMA was barred by the Seal program. What could be simpler than to cut the Gordian knot, abolish the program, and with one bold stroke cure all these financial ills? The zeal which had in the past generated consecration, crusading, and consistent pressure was gone, the cash drawer was low and might get lower. And so the club was thrown away.

The other major shift in AMA policy was in its attitude toward government regulation of drugs. It had campaigned vigorously for the first Food and Drug Law of 1908. During the next three decades relationships between the AMA and the federal agencies regulating drugs remained close. The AMA and the Bureau of Chemistry of the Department of Agriculture advanced toward a common goal by a series of lateral passes. They kept each other informed of proposed or desired legislation and lobbied for it side by side. Wiley spoke and Simmons editorialized against the same quack remedies. The Department of Agriculture analyzed dubious drugs for the AMA, and the AMA rounded up consultants for the Bureau of Chemistry.[7]

When it became obvious that a new law was needed, the AMA rallied to the support of the friends of food and drug legislation. It wanted stronger bills than those presented in Congress and even complained that one bill had been subjected to "plastic surgery in the legislative operating rooms" until it had become "an asthenic, chinless and impotent monstrosity." Even when the 1938 bill was finally passed, the AMA complained because the Department of Agriculture was given no control over the advertising of drugs to physicians.[8]

The Council on Pharmacy and Chemistry continued to cooperate with the Department of Agriculture's successor, the federal Food and Drug Administration. It is also of interest that at least two secretaries of the Council were recruited from the FDA during the 1940's, and the staffs of the two organizations collaborated on an article explaining how drugs should be tested.[9]

As late as 1953 the AMA apparently approved of stronger regulation by the FDA, because it originated a bill, eventually passed, which authorized the FDA to inspect pharmaceutical laboratories without first obtaining permission from the proprietors.[10] Yet six years later, when Senator Kefauver began his hearings on the prices of drugs and the practices of the drug industry, the AMA was lined up solidly with that industry and against the proposals for a change in the laws. The provision that the drug manufacturer had to prove his claims of efficacy before he could market a drug drew fire from the AMA because "A drug's efficacy varies from patient to patient . . . . Hence any judgment concerning this factor can only be made by the individual physician who is using the drug to treat an individual patient."[11] This was patently at variance with a statement approved by the Board of Trustees in 1954 which said, "The average physician has neither the time nor the facilities to experiment with new drugs in order to determine their proper indications for use . . . ."[12]

The AMA also opposed the portion of the proposed law which required that the Secretary of Health, Education, and Welfare determine

7. James G. Burrow, *AMA: Voice of American Medicine* (Baltimore: Johns Hopkins Press, 1963), pp. 117–18.
8. "Federal Food and Drug Bill Advanced," *JAMA* 110 (April 23, 1938): 1370–72.
9. W. Van Winkle, Jr., R. P. Herwick, H. O. Calvery, and A. Smith, "Laboratory and Clinical Appraisal of New Drugs," *JAMA* 126 (Dec. 9, 1944): 958–61.
10. U.S. Congress, *Drug Industry Antitrust Act*, pt. 2, p. 999.
11. *Ibid.*, p. 1010.
12. "Reports of Officers," *JAMA* 156 (Nov. 6, 1954): 968.

whether the therapeutic effect of a modification of a drug for which a patent application had been made was significantly greater than that of the drug so modified.[13] This position, too, disagreed with a statement of the Board of Trustees in 1920, complaining that "the profits to be made from the sale of a proprietary medicine on which the manufacturer holds a monopoly are usually large—sometimes enormous,"[14] and with the AMA's opposition to granting the Bayer Company a renewal of the patent on aspirin in 1917. Regarding the latter, the AMA stated that "practically no other country in the world . . . would grant a patent on either acetylsalicylic acid, the product, or on the process for making that product. The United States granted both!"[15]

The abandonment of the Seal program was followed by an avalanche of advertising revenue for the AMA. In 1966 the total income was nearly $28,000,000, and of this over $13,000,000, or 48 per cent, came from advertising.[16] Whether as a result of this, or because the scarcity of physicians and general prosperity had kept doctors' incomes at a high level for several decades, the AMA had moved far to the right politically since the 1920's.

The AMA changed its attitude toward compulsory health insurance from exploratory interest to violent hostility between 1917 and 1920.[17] The battle was fought in the press, in the hustings, and in the halls of Congress for several decades; it was highlighted by the prosecution of the AMA under the Antitrust Laws in 1938 and reached its high-water mark recently with the passage of Medicare.[18] It was only human, therefore, that while the AMA and one branch of the federal government were locked in a violent struggle which the AMA believed would decide whether American medicine was to survive, the AMA should suspect the motives of other government agencies. To turn the other cheek toward the FDA after being slapped by others in the federal government was more than the doctors could do; the best their spokesmen could manage was to present a polite but frosty mien when it was necessary to meet on professional matters.

What of the Future?

The missions of a quasi-official agency—one that performs a public function even though it is not directed by the people to do so—are (1)

13. U.S. Congress, *Drug Industry Antitrust Act*, pt. 2, p. 1009.
14. "Proceedings of the New Orleans Session . . . April 26–30, 1920," *JAMA* 74 (May 1, 1920): 1235.
15. Burrow, *AMA*, p. 128.
16. "AMAgrams," *JAMA* 201 (Sept. 4, 1967): adv. p. 9.
17. Burrow, *AMA*, pp. 146–51.
18. Richard Harris, "Annals of Legislation: Medicare, II; More Than a Lot of Statistics," *The New Yorker*, July 9, 1966, pp. 30–38, 41–44, 55–77.

exploratory—to experiment with new methods, to demonstrate their effectiveness, and then to turn them over to governmental units for complete implementation; (2) cooperative—to collaborate and inter-digitate with governmental agencies; and (3) supportive—to stimulate, encourage, champion the cause of, and, if necessary, watch over, public agencies so that they perform in the public interest. The AMA has accom-plished some of these objectives and failed in others.

First, it explored new areas that were eventually incorporated into the Acts of 1938 and 1962. The effectiveness of the Council on Pharmacy and Chemistry in identifying secret formulas, encouraging testing of drugs, and publicizing deleterious effects paved the way for the Food and Drug Act of 1938, which required the safety of a drug to be proved before it could be marketed. Likewise, the Council's insistence upon valid evi-dence of a drug's efficacy demonstrated the need for, and the methodology of, these evaluations, so that when the Council dropped its Seal of Accep-tance program the federal government picked it up in a more comprehen-sive form after the Kefauver-Harris Amendments of 1962.

Second, collaboration between the Council on Drugs and the FDA and their predecessors was at one time open, friendly, free, and productive. The olive branches have withered of late—to the detriment of both parties. Yet they can cooperate effectively, as shown by their success in one area, the naming of drugs.

In its supportive mission the AMA has changed directions. It en-couraged and supported the federal government in the regulation of drugs up to the 1950's. Since then, it has opposed as often as it has sup-ported, and criticized more often than it has praised.

In the future, in its exploratory function the American Medical Association might experiment with programs for reporting reactions of drugs in smaller hospitals, might study how doctors decide what drugs to give, and might encourage and certify training for doctors who test drugs.

Opportunities for collaboration are also abundant. Members of the staff of the FDA should be on the Council on Drugs; and members of the Council and the staff of the AMA should serve on advisory com-mittees of the FDA. The AMA might set up panels of experts who would be available to the FDA to give advice on particular classes of drugs. The fact that the Commissioner of Food and Drugs chose to ask the National Research Council to evaluate the efficacy of drugs that had been approved between the 1938 and 1962 Acts points up the need for the government to turn to a responsible public agency for such advice.

In its supportive function the American Medical Association can report on the relative efficacy of drugs—something the FDA is forbidden to do by law. Thus, the American Medical Association can expand and enrich the work of the Food and Drug Administration. The AMA can tackle the problem of mixtures now that the FDA is passing upon the effectiveness of single-entity drugs. We badly need a crusade against the irrational and potentially harmful mixtures that are on the market.

Finally, the AMA should ask itself why it does not support the FDA more strongly. Facts force the neutral observer to conclude that the AMA has swung around 180 degrees from being the champion of the consumer of drugs to being the champion of the drug industry. Undoubtedly the drug industry's interests do need defending; no governmental power, no matter how well intentioned, can be allowed to move unchecked. But a multimillion dollar industry with intelligent and aggressive leaders is surely capable of defending itself. On the other hand, the consumers of drugs have few champions, and those it has are sometimes better intentioned than informed. Who can look out better for the consumer's interest in the area of drugs than the physician who is knowledgeable about drugs from his training, who sees the needs of the consumer every time he treats a patient? One of the great physicians of the nineteenth century, Rudolph Virchow, said that the physician is the natural advocate of the poor. Surely he is the natural advocate for all consumers of drugs, rich or poor.

Commentary

William B. Bean

I would like to begin my comments with two quotations. One is a quotation from an epitaph from a little English country churchyard:

Here lies the body of Mary Ann Waters,
Died of drinking Cheltenham waters,
If she had stuck to Epsom salts,
She wouldn't be lying in these here vaults.

The other is a quotation from myself: "The capacity of the human mind to deceive itself knows no limits." I have modified that when I was in a slightly more benign mood by saying that "the capacity of the human mind to deceive itself knows hardly any limits."

When we consider the enormous present-day advances in science and in medicine, the powerful drugs that are available, the tremendous therapeutic possibilities, we have to reckon also that there are equal and opposite dangers and opportunities for doing damage. Historically, the emergence of therapy—drug therapy is what we are thinking of—grew as astrology gave way to astronomy, and as alchemy gave way to chemistry. The first phase of the understanding of medicine was the identification in herbs and plants of those essences which seemed to have medicinal virtue. These have continued in every society, in every culture, as the folk remedies. We can go long beyond Withering and foxglove right up to the present day. Even within the memory of people here, at least two important drugs have come from herbs whose use was embodied in folk knowledge. One is ephedrine, from the Chinese mahuang. Dr. Chen helped work out its chemistry and pharmacology. The rauwolfia compounds from India, as far as I know, are the latest.

The general trend now is for a chemist to modify or change a molecule, perhaps only slightly, hoping that he will get at once a stronger, an even less dangerous, compound. It is usual, though, that the power of a drug carries with it almost in parallel a potential for dangerous reactions.

Dr. Dowling tells us about the shift in polarization of the American Medical Association. It is quite fascinating that in one of the earlier phases he was discussing, 75 per cent of the delegates to an American Medical Association meeting came from medical schools. Today if anyone comes from a medical school, it is not because he is in a medical school, but

132

it is because he joined a county medical society and worked his way up. The basis of the grass roots support of the AMA, and part of the reason for its strong shift to the right, are the older and more conservative members of a medical community who become delegates, elected by a constituent county or city society. To have time to do this means, usually, that one has either married a wealthy wife or has practiced successfully and accumulated enough time and money to get into higher medical politics. So it is not surprising, in fact quite otherwise, that these strong polarities of the governing bodies of American medicine—the AMA—have done precisely what Dr. Dowling told us. As they have shifted their interest from being crusaders, from being, indeed, the protectors of *the people*, to being concerned with preserving their rights and the status quo, their relation with those making a living in the manufacture, distribution, and sale of drugs has gone from caution to wholesale and sometimes uncritical acceptance. It is unreasonable to suppose that anybody in a business such as the pharmaceutical industry is not interested in making money. The whole shift, then, has been from that of a careful protecting overview of the world of medical practice to the orientations that were made pretty obvious in the Kefauver Committee's confrontations which occurred in Washington not so long ago.

I think it is well for us all to remember that, though we cannot have each doctor do all the testing on every patient, each person in the world is biochemically, anthropologically, genetically, and in any other way you wish individual and unique. The postulate that there is a dose, a fixed dose, of a drug which is routine for any person with a specific disease—a standard to be applied by pressing a button in a kind of therapeutic automat—is irrational. Absorption varies. Internal bodily metabolisms are different. At one end of the spectrum there are persons who react idiosyncratically or allergically to a drug. In addition there are sensitivities that exist without harming a person at all until he encounters a new biochemical agent to which he may have a violent reaction, even though the majority of people exposed to the same thing do not react in that way. After a while he may learn not to revolt against its administration. We must reject the illusion of a fixed dose; we must remember uncertain and individualistic responses to standard therapeutic measures. We have an increasing host of powerful and potent drugs which have now made therapeutic nihilism a fiction and figment. These drugs are in many instances life-saving. We could not think of the practice of medicine without their use. But in their use in the practice of medicine we should remember that they are two-edged swords that cut back at you if you are not very careful in the way you wield them. With increased potency we have increased danger. We need the monitoring of externally applied rules and the thoughtful control by the physician who is on the firing line taking care of people for whom he prescribes and to whom he gives the drugs which, properly given, moderate, abate, and sometimes cure diseases. People who are thinking in broad terms about the history of drug regulation realize that regulations are necessary if for no other reason than the great complexity and the great power both for good and evil of our marvelous drugs. The cooperation of science with the pharmaceutical industry, the practicing physician, and certainly not least the patient has enabled us to make great progress, and we must continue by using wise regulations effectively.

Commentary

John R. Lewis

Dr. Sonnedecker presented such a complete review of the different roles of the pharmacist in the development of drug controls during the nineteenth century that it requires little additional comment. I think it is significant, however, that during this period, as pointed out by Dr. Sonnedecker, "the central goal was therapeutic equivalency for all drugs used in medical care under the same name." This goal remains today, but at times it seems elusive. In spite of advances in biochemistry, pharmacology, and biopharmaceutics, many problems remain to be solved before this goal is met.

The activities of the AMA Council on Pharmacy and Chemistry as they related to drug control were given emphasis by both Dr. Burrow and Dr. Dowling. It is this subject to which I shall address most of my comments.

As usual, Dr. Dowling raised provocative points, but my consideration of certain aspects of the Council's program leads me to some views which differ from those expressed by him. During the early years of the Council's activities, its main battle was against nostrums, quackery, and pseudo-science, and, as we were told, the Council was able to claim a victory in this area by 1920. Nevertheless, the crusade against the secret remedies, or so-called patent medicines, continued.

To win its victories the Council used two principal means. One was to limit the advertising in the AMA publications to those products which met certain criteria of the Council, and the other was to publish its findings and opinions on the products examined.

The "acceptance" of a product for advertising has been referred to as a "club" which the Council used to give it strength. It has been stated here, and many times before, that when the Council discontinued its Seal of Acceptance program it lost its "club" and thus lost its strength. I submit that other factors must also be considered.

It should be mentioned that the Council's "Seal Program" was not initiated until 1929; however, earlier it had established certain rules for acceptance of advertising. These rules were modified by the Council over the years. In 1955, when the Association discontinued its Seal of Acceptance programs—for all councils, not only the Council on Pharmacy and Chemistry—the rules governing advertising were revised, but they still contain rules to restrict certain advertising. I will not discuss the details of the present principles, but with these present guides approximately 30 per cent of advertisements are rejected, and of those accepted about 75 per cent are revised before publication.

Because acceptance of a drug for advertising seems to have been such an important factor in the success of the Council's program, I was curious about the type of ads that appeared during the Seal program, and I made a cursory examination of a few issues of *JAMA* taken at random in 1948. This revealed comparatively few drug advertisements; there appeared an average of about twenty advertisements for drugs per issue. Of course, the nonaccepted products were missing, but the drugs represented did not appear to provide much information regarding the type of products accepted and not accepted. On the other hand, in 1948 there were relatively more advertisements for products other than drugs; for example, there were advertisements for several brands of cigarettes. Now, of course, the Council did not "accept" these, but the editor must have approved them. It is noteworthy that present policy prohibits advertising such products. Furthermore, I doubt whether some of the advertisements in the 1948 *JAMA* I reviewed would be acceptable today.

It should be kept in mind that nonacceptance of a product was not necessarily based on lack of therapeutic merit. For example, while thumbing through the Council's reports for 1950, I noticed that Dolophine, Lilly's brand of methadone, was not accepted for *New and Nonofficial Remedies* because the trade name suggests the therapeutic use of the product. I find it difficult to believe that this decision had a significant effect on the physician's use of this product. It is interesting, however, that the principal use of this product now is not as an analgesic, but as an antitussive. I wonder if the Council would accept it now.

Many have criticized the AMA for discontinuing its Seal programs, and some of the reasons given for this change in policy have been discussed here, but instead of accepting the reason given by Senator Kefauver, that is, that it was done to sell more advertising, I believe the Council's statement explains the real reason. In announcing discontinuation of the Seal of Acceptance program, the Council stated:

> There is an increasing demand from the medical profession in general for concise and timely reports that contain an authoritative, unbiased evaluation of new therapeutic agents. The former acceptance program of the Council served a useful purpose in this regard for many years; however, in this present era of rapid new developments in therapeutics, the work involved in processing for acceptance many different brands of a drug became cumbersome and time-consuming to the extent that physicians could no longer be provided with the type of service they desired. Consequently, termination of the seal-acceptance program became necessary in order that the Council could embark on an expanded program of operation that would be of much more interest and value to the profession.

In the early days of the Council there were many ineffective preparations and few effective ones; the Council did a creditable job in exposing the worthless products, as the speakers have emphasized. However, with the tremendous changes in the drug industry, especially after World War II, the situation has been reversed, so that now there are few ineffective drugs and many effective ones. The Council's acceptance program was designed to handle the first situation, but it could not cope with the second. Thus, it became necessary for the Council to adopt a different approach to the problems; it concentrated its efforts on informing and educating the physician to select the product, from among those available, which could be expected to be of greatest benefit to his patient.

Much has been said about the Seal program as it related to the acceptance of advertising but little mention has been made of perhaps a more significant aspect of this program, namely, the publication of Council reports. In discussing the educational program of the Council, Dr. Dowling stated that "the doctors did not read what the Council said!" I must agree! According to a Council report, the average annual sales of *NNR* for the years 1923–43 was only 13,000; thus, it is apparent that not many physicians were using the Council's book under the Seal program. With this small circulation, if physicians heeded the Council's advice on drugs, and we are led to believe that they did, they must have depended on its reports in *JAMA* for their guidance. The most significant difference between the Council's reports during the Seal program and after its discontinuation was the publication of adverse reports on drugs in the former program. This difference was particularly apparent in the area of mixtures. Under the newer program the Council stated that the "Evaluation of ready-prepared mixtures of drugs for monograph description in *NNR* has been discontinued. Publication of timely information on each new compound should make it easier for the physician to judge which combinations are best suited for the individual patient on the basis of the Council's evaluation of separately available component drugs."

Experience over the past ten years and more has shown that this viewpoint was incorrect, and that this approach was not effective. This policy of the Council to ignore mixtures left the physician without a source of unbiased information about the new mixtures so vigorously promoted. The present Council is convinced, as were previous Councils, that the widespread use of mixtures of active drugs is, in many instances, not in accord with the best practice of medicine, but to the present they have not adequately informed physicians of their opinion. However, recently the Council has taken a significant step forward to correct this deficiency. During the time Dr. Dowling was its chairman, the Council decided to prepare and publish a comprehensive reference book that will include information on both old and new single-entity drugs and mixtures. Under the guidance of, and, I might add, the pressure on the staff by Dr. Dowling, plans for the book were started a few years ago. The book is now well on its way; it is being prepared through a joint effort of the Council, the staff of the AMA Department of Drugs, drug evaluators outside the Department working part-time, and many voluntary expert consultants.

Discussion

Mr. Gordon: I have a question to direct to Dr. Dowling. The question is quite short, but the introduction to the question is a bit longer. Last night I received a call from a friend of mine who told me about an article in an issue of *Look* magazine on the thalidomide cases that are coming up in Germany very soon. According to the article, so I was told, the company was well aware of the side effects of this drug while marketing it. In addition, all indications are that the company, Richardson-Merrell, which was pushing the new drug application in the United States also was aware of the side effects. I would like also to refer to MER 29, a rather interesting case of which I am sure you are all aware, where the company falsified information to both the medical profession and the Food and Drug Administration. The company, in this case also Richardson-Merrell, was subsequently found guilty of criminal violation of the Food and Drug Act. Its directions to detail men, which, incidentally, are found in the public record of the private cases against the company, show that the detail men were instructed to give false and misleading information to doctors. In addition, the company had written letters and articles and got doctors to sign them as if they were their own. Let us remember also that the Fond du Lac study, which was sponsored by the American Medical Association, indicated that the doctor receives most of his information on new drugs from the detail man and, to a lesser extent, from drug advertising. Recently, a *Canadian Medical Association Journal* article also emphasized the extreme dependence of the medical profession on detail men for their information. The question I want to ask is this: given this background, given the dependence of the medical profession on information from the drug industry, how is it possible to have good medical practice in the United States?

Dr. Dowling: In the presence of distinguished members of the legal profession, I am bold enough to quote an anecdote in which a witness was asked how long he had prepared his testimony, and I believe he answered, "All my life." I think the answer to what has been said here is that trying to improve the medical profession is what one devotes one's life to—and at the end one does not feel that one has gotten very far. However, some of the things that we and others are advocating are directed toward the ends that have been asked about.

It seems to me that some of the things which have been mentioned are beyond the purview of the medical profession, that is, the actual violations of the law, or alleged violations. There must be teeth in the law to take care of them, and these I think we now have, although perhaps not to a sufficient degree, and perhaps the laws are not sufficiently enforced to satisfy congressional committees. Nevertheless, we have a beginning in that direction, and our colleague from England tells us that in these things, for once, we are ahead of his country.

Beyond this, I feel that the organized profession, interdigitating with the government, must do certain things—some of the things that I have been advocating inside the Council on Drugs, and on the outside, for some time. I would go further and say that doctors have to regulate themselves and their conduct within their hospitals and within their county medical societies, that we must have some way of enforcing ethics on those doctors who will not conform.

Mr. Gordon: Mr. Chairman, I would like to pursue that a little further. I might mention to Dr. Dowling that the oral presentation of advertising is probably not controlled by the 1962 law. Right now it appears that neither the FDA nor any other government agency has any power or jurisdiction over the detail man or over any oral presentation. Even if it were part of the law, it would be extremely difficult to monitor these oral presentations. The question then is: would it be a good idea to eliminate oral presentations entirely; that is, just prohibit them by law? Then, at least, you would have the written presentations, which can be monitored.

Mr. Kleinfeld: It may be theoretical, but these oral presentations are covered by existing laws; there is no question about that.

Mr. Gordon: There is a question. As a matter of fact, to judge from the legal section of the Library of Congress and from other lawyers whom our Subcommittee has consulted, the predominant opinion is that you could not cover the oral presentation with any law now on the books.

Mr. Kleinfeld: I am not talking about the practicality of it, but in the past there have been criminal prosecutions of pitchmen under the Food and Drug Act. A detail man is a pitchman, and if he makes a false or misleading statement (we assume that this could be established, which is a difficult proposition) he could be convicted, as his predecessors have been, particularly since intent is not an element of the offense. Now, perhaps a congressional committee would want to pass a law saying that every detail man has to have a recording device along with him and has to present it to the Food and Drug Administration. But this problem is met by Congress, in my opinion, in existing law.

Mr. Cavers: To supplement Mr. Kleinfeld's remarks, it is, I think, significant that in civil litigation against pharmaceutical manufacturers the selling efforts of the detail men have been found to override the warnings that are included in the labeling and advertising, with the result that on occasions manufacturers have been held liable, and for quite large sums, by reason of the overenthusiasm of detail men.

Dr. Lasagna: I once made the fanciful suggestion that it might be advantageous to have detail men who were not hired by one particular firm but were actually subsidized by the profession, and who would bring to the attention of the practicing doctor advances or retrogressions in the field of therapeutics. The detail man is a very popular conveyor of information for the doctor, for reasons which are not hard to understand. The problem is: how can appropriate information on drug usage be brought to doctors by people who have less of a vested interest in pushing a given drug than does the manufacturer. The academic world and the profession itself have done precious little to keep doctors up to date on drugs. It must be remembered that if a unique drug is placed on the market—a drug which represents a very real advance in therapeutics—it is in the interest of both the medical profession and the public that information about this drug be rapidly and efficiently disseminated. At present, the drug industry does a rather good job at that level. The arguments arise when a drug is marketed that does not seem like a great advance, and may actually look like a step backward. I think the answer to Mr. Gordon's question is that all of us who are concerned with improving the practice of medicine must put our minds to finding more efficient ways of keeping doctors up to date in the field of therapeutics. I think that this burden is one that we have not shouldered in the past.

Dr. Beyer: I would like to make a number of comments. In an earlier discussion the impression was left that the *Pharmacopeia* was useful chiefly as a doorstop or as something to put children on when they wanted to reach the counter for a soda. I was reminded of a little monograph that was put out by the AMA back in my graduate student days, before the *NNR*, called *Useful Drugs*, which I thought was pretty good, but which, in the medical school, was promptly dubbed "Useless Drugs." This gets back to the agnostic outlook that Dr. Bean referred to, and I was delighted when he said that this attitude is inappropriate today, that there are drugs that are useful.

When a new drug comes along, it goes through three phases. If it is active, the first phase is one of enthusiasm in the company and in most of the investigators who have looked at it. It shows through in the promotion, sometimes to the embarrassment, in retrospect, of the company. But then, if another investigator is going to publish on this drug and if his publications are going to receive some recognition—or if *he* is—he has to write something new about it. So usually the second phase is a rash of publications that relate to the side effects of that drug. Then comes the third phase, when the drug settles down. It may be accepted or rejected, or it may fall somewhere in between—and not always where it should fall. This lesson I learned a long time ago when we were working with probenecid with the idea of using it with penicillin orally to get substantial blood levels with a bactericidal as well as a bacteriostatic effect. This happened to hit the market about the same time as the penicillin-beeswax combinations. The physician could understand these latter simple formulations, but the fact that one could safely inhibit the renal tubular secretion of a compound was not acceptable at that time; physicians just did not know what those renal tubules were for and could not accept the concept of the physiological economy of penicillin. To be sure, they had been using mercurial diuretics, which inhibit tubular reabsorption of salt and water, but they were getting an increase in urine flow from the diuretic, so this was good.

There was another side of the probenecid story that concerned advertising. In the early days of that compound, which was obviously useful as a uricosuric agent in gout, gout was infrequently diagnosed in this country and almost never on the Continent. Today gout is much better recognized than it was. I think the fact that there is a form of therapy available has brought into focus this entity, which was ofttimes, perhaps, misdiagnosed as some other form of arthritis. This I think indicates that there is some good in promotion and some in teaching both by professors and by the pharmaceutical industry.

Finally, in relation to Dr. Bean's comment on potency, we can say, to be sure, that as more potent compounds come along they carry with them a need for understanding. Here again, education is tremendously important. I hope that Dr. Bean will find another analogy beside that of a "two-edged sword" for increased efficacy and potency, because the idiosyncratic aspects of side effects do not relate to potency.

Dr. Bean: Change that to the "sword of Damocles"!

Dr. Beyer: The second point I would make is that, when we are using those potent compounds for lifesaving measures, the propensity of the compound to produce damage is directly related to the need for the agent. Let me say it differently. The homeostatic mechanisms in the mild to moderately ill patient are in pretty good shape. As he becomes more seriously ill, he has less control over his homeostasis. It is at this point that the physician takes over, so to speak, with the more potent medication. It is when the patient needs it most that the physician can get in the greatest trouble with new therapy. So, believe me, I am interested in the education of the physician.

Dr. Whittet: May I have a word, Mr. Chairman, as some of our experience may be interesting to you? In Britain the detail man is being overtaken by a publication called *MIMS*, the *Monthly Index of Medical Specialities*. Someone had the idea of listing every preparation on the market in Britain in a monthly throwaway edition which is sent free to all physicians. Much prescribing is done from this: in an article, it was shown that it is more widely used than the detail man. It is a private publication, supported by advertising.

I was very interested in Dr. Lasagna's comment that there should be independent detail men, because the Sainsbury Report suggested that we should have Ministry detail men to promote generics. We have tried to get advice through, first of all, the Cohen committee, which classified drugs into acceptable, less acceptable, and not acceptable. This was succeeded by the Macgregor committee, a committee on classification of drugs, which is going into this in even more detail. The trouble with these committees is that their reports are put out in Ministry White Papers, and physicians hardly ever read them. So Professor Macgregor is now trying to compete with *MIMS*, and he puts the reports out in a rather glossy form—very like *MIMS*—called "Proplist" (Proprietary Drugs List). These, we are hoping, will become more popular. We have one other educative medium, the *Prescribers' Journal*, which is, at the moment, a bimonthly journal—we hope it will be a monthly one eventually—and this publishes appraisals of drugs by experts in various fields. The governing board is entirely independent, but the secretariat is paid for by the Ministry. Actually, Dr. Lasagna has contributed an article on analgesics to the *Journal*.

Dr. Lasagna: I wonder if anyone can give us any historical insight into the origin of that interesting notion that the name of a drug should not tell what the drug does. I would have thought that the ideal name for a drug was one which told both what it did and something about its chemical structure. Was the idea that it gave unfair economic advantage to the manufacturer who was bright enough to think of a name that actually told what the drug did, or was it a belief that, in fact, the drug really did not do what the name implied?

Dr. Bean: Maybe the doctrine of signatures, having gone out of fashion, should go out of existence.

Mr. Cowen: It may have been a movement away from patent medicines, which in the nineteenth century bore such names as "Nervine" and "Brainene," but I do not know.

Dr. Lasagna: I notice of late that we seem to have dropped that notion. We now have a number of important drugs on the market whose trade names indicate quite clearly what they do.

Dr. Dowling: This was never true of trade names. The AMA Council did not attempt to stop trade names from relating to the action of the drug: it was the official name—or the name the Council hoped would be official if the *USP* took it up—although this was allowed in some instances, for example, ascorbic acid, in this case because the originator insisted that "ascorbic" be used instead of "cevitamic." I think the reason was that the Council felt that names that indicated a therapeutic action would make for sloppy practice, that is, the doctor would say, "This is what this drug is for; I'll use it." He would not look it up. It would have been something like the working mechanism that we are decrying now in advertisements. And because of this, they felt that the official name should never indicate use.

There was one other reason. Sometimes, as you know, a side reaction turns out to be a therapeutic reaction, and as a consequence the drug would have been named for one type of reaction and the doctor might be using it for something quite different. The drug we were talking about a minute ago, which Dr. Beyer had a big hand in developing, is a good example. It is used now much more for gout than it is for the inhibition of secretion of penicillin.

Dr. Lasagna: I thought Dr. Lewis's example was a trade name, though.

Dr. Lewis: Yes, that is correct, the example is Dolophine. I do not know the background for the Council's rule that it would not accept such a name for inclusion in *NNR*.

Dr. Dowling: The Council would not allow a trade name to be used except by the originating firm. I believe there was a Donnybrook because Lilly had done a lot in the development of insulin, although of course they had not discovered it, and they wanted to use "Iletin," which was their trade name. They were not allowed to do so, because the Council decided that they had not done enough to develop it, or they had not done the primary work.

In general, however, if a company did the primary work, the Council, at a certain time, would allow its trade name to be used. This is very similar to the situation now in Denmark and in Holland, where only one trade name is allowed by law, and I testified before Senator Kefauver's committee that I thought this might solve the patent question. If the originating company was allowed to use a trademark and all others had to use the pharmacopoeial name, then the doctor would have to remember only two names, and the company that had put in the original investment would collect. Nothing ever came of that suggestion in this country. Of course, it is not too late!

Part IV: Federal Regulation

Drugs and the 1906 Law

James Harvey Young

The name of the 1906 law was the Pure Food and Drugs Act; food came first, drugs second. The two had already been paired in this order in earlier bills. This ranking was doubtless implicit in the nature of things, for food is the staff of life, drugs merely the crutch. At any rate, much of the early pressure, and strong continuing support, for a law came from agrarian states. Paddock, whose bill passed the Senate in 1892, represented Nebraska, and in the final stages before enactment, leading proponents of regulation included McCumber of North Dakota, Heyburn of Idaho, Hepburn of Iowa, and Mann of Illinois. All along, the heavy balance of attention in congressional hearings and congressional debate leaned toward food abuses.

Harvey Washington Wiley, the single most significant figure in the long struggle to secure the law, worried about the nation's food. Born on an Indiana farm, Wiley had studied food analysis briefly at the German governmental laboratories in Berlin. From the Department of Agriculture, as chief chemist, Wiley launched his telling study of adulteration. Bulletin 13, begun in 1883 and continuing seriatim for sixteen years, through 1,400 pages, dealt exclusively with food, even though Congress, in authorizing the research, had included drug adulteration as a possible field of inquiry. When Wiley desired some data on drug adulteration in 1892, he had to seek it outside his own department. As late as 1903 Wiley knew little about the adulteration of drugs, having to pose questions on this subject to his aides. In Oscar E. Anderson's excellent biography of Wiley, there is a bare handful of references to drugs, except for patent medicines.

This is not to say, of course, that Wiley was wholly indifferent to drug adulteration. It is merely to emphasize his overwhelming preoccupation with the evils afflicting America's food supply. This preoccupation carried over into Wiley's enforcement policies between 1907, when the Pure Food and Drugs Act became effective, and 1912, when he resigned. His energies during these years went primarily toward combating unclean and sophisticated food and drink—milk, eggs, poultry, oysters, wheat, vinegar, wine, whiskey, and processed foods containing chemical preservatives. This last category Wiley did consider "drugged." Adding chemicals like boric, salicylic, and benzoic acids to foods he deemed both deceptive

147

and, on the basis of his "Poison Squad" experiments, dangerous to health. A catsup maker once told a congressional committee that raw cranberries contained a higher proportion of benzoic acid than the packers wanted to put in catsup. "It seems to me," the packer said, "that if the Almighty put it there, the manufacturer ought to be allowed to use it." Wiley answered that cranberries would be more wholesome had the Almighty left benzoic acid out. Such chemicals, added to food, Wiley opposed with his most fervent passion, and controversies stemming from this stand caused the chief chemist his greatest difficulties, both with industry and with his administrative superiors, and led directly to his resignation. More than three quarters of the Bureau of Chemistry's first 1,000 Notices of Judgment, reporting terminated cases under the law up to August, 1911, were in the food field. Less than a quarter related to drugs.

The majority of the drug Notices of Judgment concerned patent medicines. Shortly before the passage of the 1906 law, nostrums had come to seem the most threatening menace in the field of drugs. Perceptive physicians and pharmacists had long opposed them. State chemists had analyzed them and revealed the shocking disparity between the therapeutic claims made on their labels and the therapeutic power—or lack of it—in their ingredients. The American Medical Association, engaged in a general housecleaning, had become exercised about the patent medicine evil, especially those nostrums promoted to physicians. Muckrakers like Samuel Hopkins Adams had sounded the alarm to the general public. Wiley himself had been moved by these events. In 1903 he had begun to make antinostrum speeches and to suggest that the drug definition in the pending law should be broadened to cover proprietary remedies. That same year a drug laboratory was set up in Wiley's Bureau. Patent medicines joined catsup and whiskey as a theme for congressional debate.

The 1906 law was drafted to define "drug" in a broad way, to include "any substance or mixture of substances intended to be used for the cure, mitigation, or prevention of disease." Misbranding under the law covered "any statement, design, or device [on the label] regarding . . . [a drug], or the ingredients or substances contained therein, which shall be false or misleading in any particular." For a short list of drugs considered especially dangerous—alcohol, morphine, opium, cocaine, heroin, alpha- or beta-eucaine, chloroform, cannabis indica, chloral hydrate, and acetanilid—the law required that the label state the proportion or the quantity contained in the medicine.

Although Wiley and his colleagues put major stress on seeking to clean up the nation's food supply, they devoted some attention to patent medicine abuses. In the first contested criminal prosecution under the law, the Bureau acted against the maker of a headache mixture loaded with acetanilid with the beguiling name of Cuforhedake Brane-Fude. The case was won. President Theodore Roosevelt urged the District Attorney to urge the judge to send the manufacturer to jail. But only a fine was assessed.

Many other headache "cures" were prosecuted. Campaigns were also launched against broad-gauge tonics with panacea claims (one was Humbug Oil), against male-weakness remedies (like Sporty Days Invigorator), and against alleged "cures" for narcotic addiction, cancer, and other dread diseases. Most proprietors, when haled into court, did not contest the misbranding charges, but paid their modest fines, modified their labels slightly, continued their earlier claims in advertising (which the law in no way circumscribed), and went on about their profitable businesses. Out in Kansas City, one proprietor resisted. An Eclectic physician, he vended an assortment of tablets and liquids as "Dr. Johnson's Mild Combination Treatment for Cancer," claiming on his label that it would produce a cure. When the government charged that this claim was "false and misleading," Johnson replied that the government had no case, arguing that the law's taboo on false and misleading statements was not intended to apply to therapeutic claims. In due course the Supreme Court agreed with him.

This decision, wrote the incensed journalist George Creel, provided "first aid to fraud and murder," leaving the nostrum provisions of the law with "as much bite as a canton flannel dog." Asking Congress to plug the hole, President Taft stated that the Johnson decision had wiped out over 150 similar cases pending in the courts, "involving some of the rankest frauds by which the American people were ever deceived." Congress quickly passed the Sherley Amendment in 1912. Devised with an eye to the Supreme Court's logic, this act banned only those therapeutic claims in patent medicine labeling that were both "false and fraudulent." Since fraudulency at law required proving a state of mind, the word "fraudulent," Wiley asserted, was a "joker" which would nullify the law's intent.

By this time Wiley was gone from the government. His successor as chief of the Bureau, Carl Alsberg, although also giving food matters the top priority, undertook a crash campaign to enforce the Sherley law. Transferring as many chemists as could be spared from other work, he had hundreds of nostrums analyzed in a short time. Many legal actions were begun. Before long, the Supreme Court gave its approval to the Sherley Amendment phrasing. Alsberg relied less on criminal prosecutions, which took much time to prepare, than on the 1906 law's other weapon, the seizure, aimed not at the maker but at the article itself. Most of the cases concerned nostrums claiming to help with diseases or conditions for which, virtually all doctors would agree, the medicines could not possibly prove of benefit: kidney and liver remedies, mineral waters sold with cure-all claims, male rejuvenators, venereal disease treatments, cancer and tuberculosis cures.

Again, victories were won. But within a decade, the Bureau encountered another stubborn antagonist, a retired court reporter who vended a liniment, made of turpentine, ammonia, formaldehyde, oils of mustard and wintergreen, and raw eggs, as a tuberculosis cure. Now the Sherley Amendment "joker" came into play. A jury was persuaded that the court reporter believed in the efficacy of his excoriating mixture and hence could not be guilty of fraudulent intent. Thus, while the 1906 law had done much good, especially because the major makers of proprietaries had voluntarily become more circumspect in their labeling—if not their advertising—no millennium was anywhere in sight. Loss of the liniment case in 1922 posed a drastic new threat to the modest degree of control that had been achieved.

Prescription drugs were also subject to control under the 1906 law. They received a lower priority in the enforcement effort, mainly because food and patent medicine abuses seemed more urgent public problems, and partly, perhaps, because virtual therapeutic nihilism reigned in the highest echelons of American medicine. These were the years when the Rev. Frederick T. Gates, perusing the pages of Osler's textbook, found so few truly curative drugs mentioned that he determined John D. Rockefeller should finance a research institute to do something drastic about the situation. Critics were complaining that the teaching of the materia medica in medical schools had so dwindled in emphasis that young physicians became easy prey for quack promotions. Yet even those doctors most skeptical of drug therapy prescribed some drugs, and most doctors, in the nation's yet unreformed state of medical practice, prescribed many. Ample evidence existed that many crude drugs, synthetic agents, and medicinal preparations on the market fell below official standards or their own professed standards. Abundant proof had been submitted to congressmen considering legislation from the 1880's on. One of the first tasks of the Bureau of Chemistry's drug laboratory was to survey this field: the results composed a gloomy bulletin published in 1904.

To be legal, under the 1906 law, all drugs recognized in the *United States Pharmacopoeia* and the *National Formulary* had to meet the standards of these volumes for strength, quality, and purity, as determined by the tests set forth. To this rule, however, there was an exception, the so-called variation clause, included in the law at the behest of pharmaceutical manufacturers who put out *USP* and *NF* drugs in forms of less than full strength. This was permitted as long as the label plainly stated the drug's actual standard. In drugs not covered by the two official volumes, adulteration occurred if they fell below, in strength or purity, the professed standard under which they were sold. A drug was misbranded if it was "an imitation of or offered for sale under the name of another article."

Most crude drugs came from abroad. As early as 1848 Congress had forbidden the importation of adulterated drugs, putting the responsibility for inspection on the Treasury Department. After a few years this law became moribund, since drug examiners were usually untrained political spoilsmen. With the enactment of the 1906 law, the Bureau of Chemistry assumed the task of examining drugs offered for import, rendering decisions on quality for the Treasury to enforce. The Attorney General ruled that the provisions of both the 1848 and 1906 laws were applicable.

Scores of foreign patent medicines were rejected. The initial deplorable condition of crude drugs offered for import improved considerably as the years went by. But there were frequent retrogressions and constant problems due to variations in the growing seasons, disturbance of trade conditions (especially during World War I), inadequate manpower for proper inspection, and the persistence of human cupidity. Asafetida is an example. Before the 1906 law, imported shipments often contained as much as 90 per cent foreign material. The proportion of gum resin, extracted by alcohol, fell far below the approved pharmacopoeial level. In time, a higher proportion of imports met the standards, but always some shipments required rejection. Shippers also temporarily found a way to fool examiners and analysts, adulterating with cheap foreign gums that also were soluble in alcohol. This required the Bureau to devise new and more accurate methods of testing, a necessity that arose with respect to many other crude drugs as well. Color reactions and new chemical methods to insure that the purified resin was really asafetida were developed. The Bureau's interest in this crude drug eventually declined. In 1923 the chief American processor of asafetida told a Bureau agent that most imports then coming in were of quite good quality, containing no more than 50 per cent foreign materials. A glycerated form of the drug was still being used by many druggists in preparing pills and tablets. "Certain classes of people, particularly in the South," the processor said, "use this glycerated asafetida for warding off diseases by chewing it or hanging it around their necks."

Other examples abound: senna, buchu, cubeb, saffron, henbane, and literally dozens of crude drugs. Often dirty, or wormy, or deteriorated, or mixed with parts of the plant containing no active agent, or replaced completely by a spurious species, these imports posed a constant problem. Sometimes a drug rejected at one of the main ports would show up later at a less important port where drug inspection was less stringent.

By the mid-1920's the Bureau had begun to place its main stress on medicinally important crude drugs, which, examination revealed, fell far short of the official mark. The Bureau helped develop bioassay methods for aconite, digitalis, strophanthus, squill, and ergot, methods which became official in 1926 with *USP X*. Thereafter, a careful eye was kept on these drugs. The *USP* method for ergot was soon revealed to be inadequate, and Bureau scientists developed a better one.

With respect to prescription drugs in interstate commerce, to judge by the Bureau's annual reports, until the mid-twenties efforts at control were unsystematic and sporadic. One fundamental problem was the paucity of analytical knowledge. Much research time was devoted to developing techniques for identifying and establishing the quantity of the various synthetic analgesics in headache mixtures, to discovering tests for narcotics in complex mixtures, to developing methods of identifying many essential oils, and to finding techniques for demonstrating the presence of alkaloids in complex galenicals. Even this work was delayed by the sad state of chemical reagents, which proved to be so poor in quality that the Bureau had to undertake a campaign of education among chemical manufacturers.

During the Wiley years, some two score crude drugs or their official preparations were acted against under the law, among them adulterated asafetida, colocynth, gentian, henbane, and belladonna. In one belladonna case, half of the pulverized drug proved to be ground olive pits. During Alsberg's regime an inquiry was made into the state of native crude drugs, including field investigation in southern Appalachia. Cases of substitution turned up (false unicorn root for true unicorn root, for example) and much too much earth, trash, and foreign matter were going to market in the guise of drugs. Educational information went forth from the Bureau to collectors and dealers. Standards of cleanliness were set, based on acid-insoluble ash. These standards, for the nonofficial crude drugs, were worked out in cooperation with members of the trade.

In 1912 the Bureau devoted considerable time to assessing the state of the market with respect to tablets and pills. Most of the products examined were intended as prescription wares, though it must be said that no fixed legal boundary was drawn between prescription and self-dosage medications until 1951. As in every fresh therapeutic province explored by the Bureau, conditions proved to be bad. Wide variations existed between the quantity of active ingredients declared on labels and the amount actually found by Bureau analysts. This was true of tablets containing such active principles as quinine, nitroglycerin, strychnine, Veronal, and various analgesics and narcotics, singly or in combination. Manufacturing plants were inspected and hearings held with producers. The Bureau concluded that shortages or discrepancies were seldom the result of willful intent but rather due to lax or faulty control in the process of manufacturing. Court actions ensued, and major pharmaceutical firms were not exempt. The Bureau seemed to put special stress on nitroglycerin products. The investigation of tablets received a very modest amount of attention until revived in the early 1920's.

Several other categories of prescription drugs concerned the Bureau now and again during the first decade and a half of its enforcement efforts. Worthy of mention were attempts to combat the adulteration of essential oils, especially oil of wintergreen; the beginning of a concern about cod-liver oil and products allegedly containing it; and the flurry of trouble with imported synthetic drugs, including neosalvarsan, after the outbreak of the war in Europe had disrupted the usual supply. The Bureau checked physicians' supply houses, which sold drugs to doctors who dispensed their own medications, and found numerous infractions of the law. The Bureau also sought to discover, by having commonly used prescriptions filled at every drug store in the District of Columbia, how well *USP* standards were being served, especially how quickly pharmacists were adjusting to the new standards in *USP IX* (1916). Conditions proved most discouraging. Hundreds of prosecutions could have been launched if the strict letter of the law had been followed. Instead the Bureau prosecuted only in the most flagrant cases and otherwise relied on warnings and an educational campaign. A survey in Puerto Rico revealed a similar widespread carelessness in prescription filling. Over this island and the federal District, the Bureau had authority to police the retail trade, a jurisdiction it lacked within the states. There, Bureau officials believed, the situation was just as bad. The best they could do was to turn the results of their surveys over to state and local food and drug officials.

In 1923 a marked increase in the intensity of the Bureau's drug control work began. Walter Campbell, who became acting chief upon Alsberg's resignation, reorganized and consolidated the administration of drug regulation and placed it in the hands of George Hoover, a physician and chemist, who had been with the Bureau since before the 1906 law. Hoover acknowledged frankly that up to that time food problems had held the ascendancy, that drug policing had lacked "sustained and systematic activity." "We find ourselves," he said, "in many particulars pioneering in the field. . . . This branch as a whole has not kept pace with the tendency of the times." Therefore, "In the light of medical science at the present time, especially the advancement of methods for the prevention and treatment of disease, and the more exact knowledge of the limitations of medicines, and the prevailing tendency to throw into the discard mysticism, superstition and secrecy, drug control work affords a great opportunity. . . ."

Hoover sought to take advantage of this opportunity. Now attention focused on bioassays of the potent and therapeutically important crude drugs and galenicals made from them. Similar stress was placed on bioassays to control glandular products, which were rising in importance in medical practice. A continuing program of checking anesthetics, especially ether, to improve their purity, was launched. Pharmaceutical tablets were reexamined, with special stress on those to be used for hypodermic injection. Variations ranged disturbingly far from official or declared standards: 0.01-grain nitroglycerin tablets, for example, ranged from an excess of 600 percent to a deficiency of 93 per cent.

This broader campaign with respect to prescription medication began during the Republican ascendancy. The Bureau's budget remained low, and Bureau policy was inevitably influenced by the prevailing political atmosphere, which emphasized cooperation with business. Administrators also realized that many of the inadequacies which their analyses revealed resulted not from deliberate fraud but from lack of proper manufacturing controls. This lack was partly due to carelessness and to the inadequate application of available scientific knowledge. It was also due to gaps in scientific knowledge or in the refinement of technological processes. Research among pharmaceutical manufacturers, one commentator stated, had been a matter for jest a mere generation earlier, and, despite activity by the two major trade associations, industrial research had not yet passed adolescence.

In view of these factors, Bureau efforts to improve the state of pharmaceuticals, while not neglecting court actions when deviation from standards was extreme, placed primary emphasis on cooperation with industry. Even with respect to Sherley Amendment enforcement involving proprietary remedies, the Bureau began the policy of warning the industry what campaigns it proposed to undertake, hoping for much voluntary reform that would curtail the scope of the legal labor needed. Much closer interaction was arranged between the Bureau and the pharmaceutical industry. Dr. Hoover spoke before the two trade associations, the American Drug Manufacturers Association and the American Pharmaceutical Manufacturers' Association. He told them frankly about the shortcomings in their wares, as revealed by the recent Bureau survey. And he besought their help. Industry could inform the Bureau, he said, what equipment it thought indispensable in a plant to assure uniform output and what degree of uniformity it was possible to achieve with the most advanced manufacturing methods and controls. Hoover also requested help from the established manufacturers in reporting the violations of the law that they encountered and in testifying for the government about trade practices when cases went to court. In turn, the Bureau would be glad to provide industry with any information it possessed which might be of value in improving standards of drug products.

Each trade association responded to Hoover's plea by appointing a contact committee to confer with Bureau officials. The first task the committees decided to confront concerned hypodermic tablets: how closely could they be made to comply with their professed standards when manufactured by the most modern techniques? In 1925 the committees had agreed on the tolerances they thought necessary even under the best manufacturing procedures. Hypodermic tablets purporting to contain 0.25 grain or more of strychnine sulfate, for example, should be permitted to vary 7.5 per cent above or below the professed quantity. Tablets purporting to contain less than 0.25 grain should be permitted a variation of 9 per cent. The Bureau wrote the contact committees' recommendations into official policy. This "advisory-before-the-act" cooperation continued. Soon after he became chief of the Food, Drug, and Insecticide Administration, which assumed the old Bureau of Chemistry's regulatory functions in 1927, Walter Campbell said that the contact committees had "contributed greatly by their activities in securing intelligent compliance with the requirements of the law on the part of the members of these [trade] associations."

One other important result of cooperation was the abandonment by pharmaceutical manufacturers of misleading drug names. Many therapeutic wares had gone forth to the prescription market called "liver stimulant," "heart remedy," "indigestion tablets," and so on. Manufacturers voluntarily modified their labels and catalogues to designate these products by composition rather than by disease condition. These revisions, the FDA asserted, had "been of great assistance in connection with the consideration of proprietary preparations of similar compositions, by removing the excuse that similar unwarranted titles . . . [were] being used by the pharmaceutical manufacturers."

The advent of the Great Depression, of course, changed many things. Sharpened competition in a falling market lowered the level of business ethics. "Completed regulatory projects are rare," Walter Campbell said in 1930. "Forms of violations apparently checked have a disconcerting habit of reappearing and calling for renewed regulatory activity." The intensification of disreputable practices was most marked in the promotion of proprietaries, but the prescription drug field was not immune. Extensive FDA surveys of *USP* and *NF* products in 1933 and again in 1936 revealed that one-eighth of all samples examined did not meet the mark. One pharmaceutical manufacturer was found to be making nitroglycerin tablets not from nitroglycerin purified for drug purposes but from plain dynamite. The tablets contained about three times as much ammonium nitrate as they did nitroglycerin. The scope of legal actions expanded because another change wrought by worsening depression conditions was a steady increase in Food and Drug Administration appropriations. All the old drug categories were policed, and new developments brought new spheres for regulation. Vitamins required increasing attention, as did the cleanliness of ampules for intravenous injection. Catgut sutures, bandages, adhesive tape, and absorbent cotton were examined for sterility. When an appellate court held that gauze bandages were "drugs" under the law, the FDA, expanding this logic and joining a national campaign to control venereal disease, attacked defective contraceptives.

The depression also brought, in time, a marked change in the psychological climate in which businessmen and bureaucrats operated. Cooperation did not cease, but relations became cooler. The situation went "so far beyond the boundaries of what we dreamed to be a possibility six months ago," wrote Charles Crawford, in charge of enforcement for the FDA, in August, 1933, "that it does not seem possible. Perhaps I have not oriented myself to the tempo of the 'new deal.'"

The situation that had changed did not include only the freedom to engage in tougher enforcement without the diplomatic necessity of first touching all the bases of industry collaboration. It also meant that a general revision of the 1906 law, to remedy weaknesses which experience had revealed, might well be possible. Indeed, after five years of struggle and compromise, that new law came.

The securing of the 1938 law is a story in its own right, too long and tortuous for telling now. One major point about prescription drugs certainly deserves mention. The 1938 law was to contain a crucial new section which regulatory officials had not sought to secure in their early drafts beginning in 1933. This last-minute section was the one giving the Food and Drug Administration responsibility for seeing that new drugs introduced into the market place be safe. A major tragedy in 1937 directly caused the presence of this clause in the law—the more than 100 deaths from diethylene glycol used by one manufacturer as a solvent for sulfanilamide. The disaster thus has a real and also a symbolical significance. If it was the poisonous solvent that moved Congress to act, it was the sulfa that heralded the whole host of chemotherapeutic agents in whose admission to the therapeutic arsenal the "new drug" clause was destined to play so indispensable a role.

Sources

For the early part of this paper, I rely on my research for *The Toadstool Millionaires* (Princeton: Princeton University Press, 1961), and on Oscar E. Anderson, Jr., *The Health of a Nation, Harvey W. Wiley and the Fight for Pure Food* (Chicago: University of Chicago Press, 1958). For the proprietary medicine discussion, I summarize material from my book *The Medical Messiahs* (Princeton: Princeton University Press, 1967). For the prescription drug section, the major sources are the annual reports of the Bureau of Chemistry and the Food and Drug Administration, as conveniently reproduced in the Food Law Institute Series volume, *Federal Food, Drug and Cosmetic Law: Administrative Reports, 1907–1949* (Chicago: Commerce Clearing House, 1951); *Food and Drug Review,* a house organ of restricted circulation begun by the Bureau of Chemistry in 1917; *Index to Notices of Judgment 1 to 10,000* (Washington, [1922?]); *Food and Drugs Act Notices of Judgment, Index to Nos. 10001–20000* (Washington, [1936?]); and a series of articles by James C. Munch and James C. Munch, Jr., "Notices of Judgment," in *Food Drug Cosmet. Law J.* 10 (1955): 219–42, and 11 (1956): 17–34 and 196–211. The generalizations made here with respect to prescription drugs will be further tested by research now under way in primary materials in the Food and Drug Administration archives.

The Evolution of the Contemporary System of Drug Regulation under the 1938 Act

David F. Cavers

In the early 1930's drug control seemed essentially a problem of how best to protect the public against quacks. A major objective then was to remove the barrier to successful prosecution erected by the Sherley Amendment's requirement that, to establish misbranding, drug claims had to be proved "false and fraudulent."[1] Another important, if lesser, objective was to provide against the sale of drugs that were "dangerous" as used and also to require that the drug's labeling contain adequate directions for use.[2]

It was only when the 1938 Act was approaching passage that the sulfonamides were introduced, a development of historic importance in the evolution of drug control, both at the time and over the succeeding quarter century. Their immediate role in drug control was to trigger the Elixir Sulfanilamide tragedy[3] and thus to provide a stimulus for creating an administrative procedure for the premarketing clearance of new drugs of uncertain safety. But the sulfonamides heralded the revolution in drugs that took place during the period covered by this paper, the twenty-four years from the 1938 Act to the Kefauver-Harris Amendments of 1962.[4] How did that revolution affect drug regulation, the attitudes

---

1. The Amendment was passed to counteract *Johnson* v. *United States*, 221 U.S. 488 (1911), in which the Supreme Court, *per* Holmes, J., held the 1906 Act's misbranding provision not to apply to therapeutic claims. Proof of fraudulent intent to satisfy the Amendment's second criterion necessitated protracted trials to convict vendors of worthless nostrums. See Young, The Medical Messiahs, cc. 3, 5 (1967). The 1938 Act returned to the 1906 Act's language, "false or misleading in any particular," for its definition of misbranding. See Food, Drug and Cosmetic Act, 52 Stat. 1040 (June 25, 1938), §502(a), 21 U.S.C. §352(a). (Hereafter cited as "FDC Act.") The Act also specified that a representation might be misleading by reason of the omission of material facts. §201(n), 21 U.S.C. §32(n).
2. See FDC Act, §502(j), 21 U.S.C. §352(j) ("dangerous to health when used in the dosage, or with the frequency or duration prescribed, recommended, or suggested in the labeling thereof"); §502(f) (1), 21 U.S.C. §352(f) (1) ("adequate directions for use").
3. The untested use of diethylene glycol as a solvent for sulfanilamide killed over 100 persons. For the official report, see Sen. Doc. 124, 75th Cong., 2nd sess. (1937), reprinted in Dunn, Federal Food, Drug and, Cosmetic Act, App. F, p. 1316 (1938).
4. Pub. L. No. 87–781, 76 Stat. 780 (Oct. 10, 1962).

toward it in Congress, and the response to it of the affected professions and industries? What adaptations did this revolution require in the machinery of drug control?

The apparatus for new drug control which, without hearings, the Congress hurried into the 1938 Act was then viewed less as the means of equipping the government to cope with a rising tide of new and hazardous drugs and more as a means of preventing the marketing of untested, potentially harmful drugs, not generally recognized as safe by experts qualified to make such judgments. Section 505 of the new Act sought to do this by forbidding such "new drugs" to be introduced in interstate commerce unless the Food and Drug Administration (FDA) had found that the sponsor's new drug application—his "n.d.a."—satisfied certain regulatory specifications.[5] If it did, the application "became effective," a phrase borrowed from the Securities Act enacted five years earlier. Under the Securities Act, a registration statement "became effective" once the Securities and Exchange Commission was satisfied that it complied with the Act.[6] This language had the further virtue of avoiding the appearance of licensing or of official approval.

I shall postpone further discussion of the evolution of new drug controls until later in this paper. First I must report briefly the impact of another drug development of great importance, one that disclosed the limitations of §505 machinery. This was no less than the first antibiotic, penicillin. Accurately stating the claims for this miracle drug could not assure its safety in use; its quality had to be established batch by batch. This was provided for by a 1945 amendment, adding a new §507 that not only subjected the antibiotic to batch certification but also set up other control procedures resembling those in §505.[7] Two years later streptomycin was brought under §507,[8] and, four years later, chlortetracycline, chloramphenicol, and bacitracin.[9] These five antibiotics continued to be the sole objects of this type of surveillance until in 1962 the Section's reach was extended to all antibiotics.[10]

5. FDC Act, §505, 21 U.S.C. §355. Perhaps the most important requirement was the submission of "full reports of investigations which have been made to show whether or not such drug is safe for use." Id. §505(b) (1), 21 U.S.C. §355(b) (1).

6. Securities Act of 1933, §8, 15 U.S.C. §77(h). In the absence of action by the Securities and Exchange Commission to the contrary, a registration statement becomes effective twenty days after filing "or such earlier date as the Commission may determine."

7. FDC Act, §507, 21 U.S.C. §357, as added by Act of July 6, 1945, c. 281, §3, 59 Stat. 463. Limitations of space have led me to omit from the text mention of the provision for the certification of drugs containing insulin, a provision added in 1941. FDC Act, §506, 21 U.S.C. §356.

8. 61 Stat. 11 (1947), amending FDC Act, §507, 21 U.S.C. §357.

9. 63 Stat. 409 (1949), amending FDC Act, §507, 21 U.S.C. §357.

10. As amended in 1962, *supra* note 4, the FDC Act, §507(a), 21 U.S.C. §357(a), now adds, after the original five: "any other antibiotic drug, or any derivative thereof."

The Control of Prescription Drugs

At this juncture I wish to direct your attention to an obscure proviso in the 1938 Act that was destined to be the starting point for some of the most potent controls the FDA exercises in the drug field today. This was simply the power to exempt by regulation drugs from the requirement in §502 (f)(1) that their labeling give adequate directions for use.[11]

The chief consequence of this exempting power was the emergence of the prescription drug as the object of special controls. The need to provide labeling directions, obvious enough for over-the-counter or "o-t-c" drugs, seemed not only superfluous in the case of prescription drugs but even hazardous. Therefore, the exempting regulation required that prescription drugs carry only the legend: "Caution: to be used only by or on the prescription of a physician," or other licensed practitioner.[12] However, to police this requirement, FDA's control had to extend to the retail druggist. This survived challenge, on constitutional and statutory grounds, in *United States* v. *Sullivan*, where the Supreme Court upheld the conviction of a retail druggist in Columbus, Georgia, who had sold over his counter a prescription drug—sulfathiazole—in an inadequately labeled bottle.[13]

With the FDA's power over prescription drugs established and their numbers expanding, the adequacy of FDA regulations as a means of designating drugs in this category came into question. How was the pharmacist to identify a prescription drug?

Though the regulations did define prescription drugs, drug manufacturers did not apply the concept uniformly. A drug would be categorized as an o-t-c drug by one pharmaceutical house and as a prescription drug by another. With the *Sullivan* case as a warning, retail druggists were concerned by the risk of criminal liability for selling over the counter what they should have dispensed only on prescription. Moreover, they had been vexed by the FDA's interpretation of the Act's requirement that all prescriptions be in writing as extending to refills, that prescriptions were to be as nonrefillable as a bank check.[14]

This mounting tension led to a major amendment to the Food, Drug, and Cosmetic Act in 1951: the Humphrey-Durham Amendment[15]

11. The authority is contained in a proviso authorizing exemptions from any requirement "not necessary for the protection of public health."
12. See 21 Code of Federal Regulations, Cum. Supp. June 2, 1938–June 1, 1943, Bk. 4, §2.107. (Hereafter cited as "CFR.")
13. *United States* v. *Sullivan*, 332 U.S. 689 (1948).
14. See Statement of R. S. Warnack, retail druggist, Los Angeles, California, Hearings on H.R. 3298 before the House Committee on Interstate and Foreign Commerce, 82nd Cong., 1st sess. (May 1–5, 1951) at 43, 48–49, complaining of speech by Food and Drug Commissioner Dunbar.
15. 65 Stat. 648 (1951), FDC Act, §503(b), 21 U.S.C. 353(b).

setting up prescription drugs as a special statutory category comprising three subcategories: A—drugs required by §502(d) of the Act to be labeled, "Warning: May be habit forming"; B—drugs which, because of toxicity or other dangers in substance or mode of use, were unsafe unless administered by a licensed practitioner; and C—new drugs limited by the terms of an effective §505 application to use under similar supervision.[16] The Amendment also included two essentially noncontroversial provisions, strongly supported by retail druggists: (1) an authorization to the physician to give prescriptions to the pharmacist orally, provided the latter made an immediate written note of the call, and (2) an authorization to refill prescriptions identified as refillable.[17] These two provisions had been overshadowed in the hearings[18] and debates[19] on the Amendments by two other issues: (1) Should the Administrator of the Federal Security Agency (FSA), of which the FDA then formed a part, determine by administrative action which drugs were to be placed in category B? (2) Should one of the criteria for placing drugs in category B be a finding that the drug is "ineffective" for use without the diagnosis or supervision of a licensed practitioner?

The Congress revealed itself as fearful of entrusting the FSA Administrator with this grant of power. Part of the fear was *ad hominem*: conservatives viewed Oscar Ewing, then Administrator, as a champion of socialized medicine.[20] To check the Administrator's power, his actions were to be subjected to judicial review *de novo*. That is, the courts were to examine the Administrator's action not on the basis of a record made before him but in a wholly new court proceeding. This was questioned as vesting legislative authority in the federal judiciary and so as going beyond their constitutional power.[21] Moreover, the review was one which obviously would be burdensome to a nonexpert tribunal. Opposition to this authority was voiced vigorously and effectively by spokesmen for

16. The statutory criteria stated above have been condensed.

17. Authority to refill may also be oral if noted in writing by the pharmacist.

18. For the House hearings, see *supra*, note 14; for the Senate hearings, see Hearings on S. 1186 and H. R. 3298 before the Subcommittee on Health of the Senate Committee on Labor and Public Welfare, 82nd Cong., 1st sess. (Sept. 11–13, 1951).

19. For the debate in the House, see 97 Cong. Rec. 9321–49 (Aug. 1, 1951). The Senate adopted the House bill with brief discussion and a few minor amendments on the floor.

20. Referring to the Administrator's power under B which his own amendment was designed to deny, Rep. O'Hara (R. Minn.) said, "Now, that is a perfectly ridiculous situation to give this tremendous power to Oscar Ewing. I like Oscar Ewing personally; I like his frankness. He is for socialized medicine. He has stated so . . . before our Committee." *Id.* at 9340.

21. See Letter of April 30, 1951, by Oscar Ewing, FSA Administrator, to Rep. Robert Crosser, Chairman, House Committee on Interstate and Foreign Commerce, H. R. Rep. No. 700, to accompany H. R. 3298, 82nd Cong., 1st sess. (1951) at 22.

the federal court system.[22] The House cut the Gordian knot by voting to abandon administrative listing and to rely simply on the statutory definition.[23] The Senate concurred.[24]

The effectiveness issue which this solution eliminated was a harbinger of issues to come. The FDA argued that, in supporting this provision, it was not concerned with a drug's effectiveness *per se* but only with its effectiveness in the absence of a physician's supervision.[25] The AMA saw the provision as encroaching on the physician's prerogatives,[26] and the drug industry viewed with alarm the combination of this provision with administrative listing of prescription drugs. An industry spokesman foretold the use of the effectiveness criterion to require a prescription as a prerequisite to obtaining a simple household remedy, aspirin, for example.[27] This same argument had been made with respect to the same drug by opponents of the Tugwell Bill's provision listing certain diseases for which the advertisement of drugs for self-medication was not to be permitted,[28] a provision that Canada took over virtually intact in 1934[29] and has lived with ever since. Canada has headaches aplenty these days, but aspirin is still sold o-t-c in Ottawa.

22. See Statement by Chief Judge Stephens of the U.S. Court of Appeals for the District of Columbia Circuit, Hearings on H.R. 3298, *supra* note 14, at 206; Letters of March 29 and April 12, 1951, by H. P. Chandler, Administrative Office of the United States Courts, to Rep. Robert Crosser, Chairman, House Committee on Interstate and Foreign Commerce, *id.* at 6–9.

23. The O'Hara amendment having this effect was carried 141 to 85. See 97 Cong. Rec. 9349 (1951).

24. See Sen. Rep. No. 946 to Accompany H.R. 3298, 82nd Cong., 1st sess., at 2. The Senate Committee stressed the Administrator's power to clarify the prescription drug category by interpretative regulations.

25. See Statement by G. P. Larrick, Assoc. Commissioner of Food and Drugs, Hearings on H.R. 3298, *supra* note 14, at 94.

26. See Statement of Dr. W. B. Martin on behalf of the American Medical Association, Hearings on S. 1186 and H.R. 3298, *supra* note 18, at 212–13, declaring the AMA to be "unalterably opposed" to provisions giving the FSA "dictatorial power to decide which drugs shall be sold on prescription," a "power to determine the therapeutic value of drugs—a decision which is a traditional and time-tested function of the medical profession." The AMA approved H.R. 3298, from which FSA's power to identify prescription drugs administratively had been deleted. See also report in House debate of vote in opposition to clause (B) by Association's board of trustees. 97 Cong. Rec. 9326 (Aug. 1, 1951).

27. See Statement of L. D. Harrop, Gen. Counsel, American Drug Manufacturers Association, Hearings on H.R. 3298, *supra* note 14, at 145.

28. This provision, §9(c) of S. 1944, 73d Cong., 1st sess. (1933), was the peg on which the aspirin charge was usually hung. For an example of the charge, see Cavers, The Food, Drug, and Cosmetic Act of 1938: Its Legislative History and Substantive Provisions, 6 Law & Contemp. Prob. 2, 10 (1939).

29. Introduced by c.54 of the Statute of Canada, 1934, amending Can. Rev. Stat. (1927) c. 76, the provision was revised somewhat in c.38 of the Statutes of Canada, 1952–53. The list of ailments for which advertising to the public was proscribed was revised by an Order in Council in May, 1967, the list being enlarged to forty-five ailments, some being eliminated and others being renamed. See 101 Can. Gazette, No. 11 (June 14, 1967).

In retrospect, the loss of this legislative battle may be viewed philosophically; it may have been one of those defeats that won a war. Administrative listing of prescription drugs, particularly when effectiveness was the ground for the need of a physician's supervision, might have evoked endless controversy, overburdening the FDA, already staggering under its workload, and perhaps discrediting for a generation the use of this form of administrative control as well as this criterion. The penalty would have been paid for a relatively small gain: the number of drugs sold over the counter would probably not have been much smaller, and the ill will engendered in the process might have blocked the far more important grant of power to evaluate the effectiveness of new drugs which was enacted a decade later.

The FDA's Relations with the Congress

During this period when the FDA was gradually developing its controls in the drug field, how was it faring in the Congress? Perhaps the best test of this is the FDA's appropriation record. This was well-nigh desperate for nearly twenty of the twenty-four years.

Taking the fiscal year (FY) 1938 as a base line, since it did not reflect the new law's demands, we find the FDA asking for, and receiving, an appropriation of $2,019,578.[30] Despite its manifold new duties, in FY 1940 the FDA was granted only $2,547,958.[31] Bearing witness to the limited scale of new drug control under §505, the amount appropriated for this was $103,000.[32]

Soon after the new act had been placed on the books came World War II. Though the FDA had to devote much manpower to aiding the armed services in meeting the many demands created by military procurement of food and drugs, its appropriation had fallen by about $100,000 by FY 1944.[33] After the war, salary and cost increases made inroads in the purchasing power of the FDA's slowly rising budget.[34]

A vivid illustration of the seriousness of its political weakness is provided by the story of the pseudo baby beets. A small businessman in

30. 50 Stat. 427 (1937). This total reflects the subtraction of $208,000 for enforcement of the Insecticide Act to make the total comparable to totals in later years when that act was not an FDA responsibility.

31. 53 Stat. 971 (1939). An adjustment has been made in this total like that reported in note 30, *supra.*

32. This figure appears as an estimate for FY 1940 in the Budget of the United States Government for the Fiscal Year Ending June 30, 1941, at 345.

33. In FY 1941, the FDA's appropriation, adjusted as in note 30, reached its prewar peak at $2,544,156. 54 Stat. 558 (1940). By FY 1944, it had fallen to $2,457,980. 57 Stat. 499 (1943).

34. Over the ten years following FY 1944, FDA's appropriations rose less than $3,000,000, standing at $5,200,000 in FY 1954.

upstate New York with more ingenuity than ethics developed a machine for carving up fully grown beets into small globes so that, when bottled, they resembled baby beets, however much they lacked the succulence of the real thing. When the FDA ruled his process in violation, this entrepreneur appealed to his congressman, who was none other than the redoubtable Representative John Taber, then the ranking Republican on the all-powerful House Appropriations Committee.

Representative Taber considered the bureaucratic assault on his constituent "about as close to an absolute outrage as" he had "ever known the Government to get into." He called Commissioner Crawford to his office and there was outraged still further when the Commissioner "insisted on his position that it violated the law," as Mr. Taber later reported to Commissioner Larrick, adding, "I had no recourse except the appropriation. . . . If you are spending a lot of money on that kind of business your appropriation ought to be cut." [35] Presumably, it was this lesson that dropped the FDA's appropriation by about $400,000, reducing it for FY 1954 to $5,200,000 from its FY 1953 level of $5,600,000. [36]

As the fifties advanced, the FDA began to feel the effects generated by increasing numbers of drug discoveries. Demands for its medical evaluations were mounting. Pharmaceutical houses and government laboratories were building up research staffs. A single drug—rauwolfia serpentina—had alone given rise to new applications from 319 different drug firms covering 2,500 different medicines. [37] A backlog of n.d.a.'s were awaiting disposition, and, of course, the FDA's troubles were not confined to drugs.

In this critical period in FDA's history, a band of rescuers was at hand. Early in 1955, Secretary Hobby of HEW (which had succeeded to FSA as FDA's departmental home) appointed a Citizens' Advisory Committee (CAC) to study the administration of the FDC Act. [38] After five months it issued a comprehensive report. It was not sensational, but its conclusions were forthright. "Although the Committee found

35. 1956 Appropriation Hearing, Departments of Labor and Health, Education and Welfare, 84th Cong., 1st sess. at 67 (Feb. 8, 1955).
36. For the appropriation for FY 1953, see 66 Stat. 362 (1952), for FY 1954, see 67 Stat. 249 (1953). The House Appropriations Committee did not relent the next year; the appropriation for FY 1955 was still lower, $5,100,000. 68 Stat. 438 (1953).
37. Commissioner G. P. Larrick, testifying in 1957 Appropriation Hearing, Departments of Labor and Health, Education and Welfare, 84th Cong., 2nd sess. at 54 (Jan. 31, 1956).
38. The Advisory Committee idea was advanced by the Department in Appropriations subcommittee hearings in the lean year of 1954, when, thanks to Rep. Taber's disciplinary budget cut, the FDA "was at a crossroads," as the Committee's report later put it. See Citizens' Advisory Committee of the Food and Drug Administration, Report to the Secretary of Health, Education, and Welfare, H. Doc. No. 227, 84th Cong., 1st sess. (June, 1955) at 3.

certain organizational and procedural weaknesses . . . ," the Report declared, "each area of the Committee's study contributed clear evidence that inadequacy of funds was the underlying cause of almost all other shortcomings." [39]

In the field of drugs, the Committee made some procedural criticisms and stressed the importance of developing research activities within FDA, not only to acquire knowledge but also to invigorate the staff and its scientific interests. The Committee even deplored the shrinkage of FDA's legal staff; its places in the Office of the General Counsel had dwindled from twenty in 1949 to twelve in 1954.[40]

Perhaps the most important of the CAC's contributions was its conception of the order of magnitude of the support required to enable the FDA to fulfill its mission to protect the American consumer. The CAC bluntly said that the FDA ought to have "a threefold to fourfold increase" in its annual operating budget "in a period of 5 to 10 years."[41]

The impact the Report had in Congress appears in the appropriations for the next three fiscal years. They rose by 10.3 per cent in FY 1957, 42 per cent in FY 1958, and 13.3 per cent in FY 1959, reaching nearly $11,000,000 in that year.[42] After five years, FDA's support was over three times its level of $5,484,000 in FY 1956 and by FY 1964 the increase had risen to $35,805,000, more than sixfold the 1956 figure.[43] The CAC's prescription had proved too modest.

The New Drug Regulations

If one pursues the new drug regulations through the *Code of Federal Regulations* and the *Federal Register*, one is struck by the continuing process of elaboration. New drug regulations first appear in the first supplement to the Code, for June, 1938, to June, 1943.[44] By the end of those five years, the Code provisions required exactly one page to cover the n.d.a. and the exemption permitting investigational drugs to be shipped in interstate commerce before their applications became effective. Plainly the regulation was then conceived chiefly as a barrier to another Elixir Sulfanilamide tragedy.

39. *Id.* at 53.
40. *Id.* at 6, 17, 55.
41. *Id.* at 5.
42. For a comparison of the funds provided the FDA, as well as its staffing and workload, for FY 1956–62, see Report of the Second Citizens' Advisory Committee on the Food and Drug Administration to the Secretary of Health, Education and Welfare, App. A, p. 90 (October, 1962).
43. For the appropriation for FY 1956, see 69 Stat. 401 (1955), for FY 1964, see 77 Stat. 229 (1963). (The FY 1956 was later supplemented by $660,000 for Salk vaccine operations and a $360,000 pay raise.)
44. 21 CFR, Cum. Supp. June 2, 1938–June 1, 1943, Bk. 4, §§2.108–2.114.

Modest additions were made in nearly every one of the ensuing years, and in 1955 a major operation, including a detailed form for applications, was proposed and, about a year later, was adopted with few changes.[45] The same regulations also prescribed procedures to govern hearings within the agency before adverse decisions were reached on n.d.a.'s.[46]

Despite this process of development, drug regulations were open until 1963 to one serious complaint: the review process in the FDA did not begin until the filing of what the applicant hoped would be the completed n.d.a. Unknown to the FDA until then were the pharmacological and clinical investigations on which the applicant was relying and the identity of the pharmacologists and clinical investigators who were to carry these out. To be sure, the drug's sponsor had to acquire from the investigators statements of the qualifications and physical equipment, if any, needed for tasks they were assuming, and these were to be kept on file for a three-year period.[47] However, there was little reason for the sponsor to expect these records to be scrutinized before the submission of his n.d.a., absent serious—and publicized—adverse reactions.

I understand that proposals to require applicants to file their investigational plans with FDA had earlier been considered in the agency, and there had received a cold response from some of those engaged in medical evaluation. If this was indeed the case, I suspect that it resulted from the reluctance of these overburdened men to expose themselves to another influx of paper, even though sometimes this examination would reveal defects in investigational plans or personnel.

Of course, more than the efficiency of the reviewing process was at stake. Badly conceived investigations or an insufficiency of animal studies could expose the patients on whom the drugs were being tried to dangers that might otherwise have been warned against. Moreover, after investigations have been completed, the temptation to accept their results, rather than to insist on new or additional work, must always be greater than at the start of the process. In any event, when in 1962 a new law was imminent, one which would require a new drug's effectiveness as well as its safety to be evaluated, the FDA proposed,[48] and soon after the law's passage adopted, an extensive addition to the new drug regulations calling for filing the claim for the investigational drug exemption, now known as the IND, containing not only investigational plans but also investigators' statements of their qualifications and their recognition of

45. For the proposed rules, see 20 Fed. Rep. 6584 (1955); for the rules as adopted, 21 CFR, Pt. 130, see 21 Fed. Reg. 5576 (1956).
46. *Id.* at 6587, 21 CFR §§130.14–130.31.
47. 21 CFR §130.3 (a)(4). This requirement dates from the first new drug regulations, *supra* note 44, §2.114 (a)(5).
48. 27 Fed. Reg. 7990 (Aug. 10, 1962).

the obligations they were assuming.[49] The FDA retained power to terminate the exemption on any one of eleven specified grounds, including findings that the investigation was not "reasonably safe," that its plan was not "reasonable," and that reports of progress or of serious hazards were not made as specified.[50]

What was the grist of this new drug application mill? In its first three years applications came in at a rate running well over 100 a month, testifying to the manufacturers' uncertainty about whether their products would be considered "new drugs" by the FDA.[51] Thereafter the inflow settled down to about 300 a year plus supplemental applications.[52] As the drug revolution began to gain momentum, however, the number of n.d.a.'s steadily rose to an average in the fifties of about 500 per year[53] and, of course, the more applications that were effective, the more supplemental applications they bred. Also, the drug revolution was not confined to drugs for the human species; in one year new veterinary drugs numbered more than new drugs intended for man.[54]

A lawyer observing this inflow might have indulged in hopeful anticipation of lawyer's work to come. If so, he was destined to disappointment. In the first nine years, of 6,264 applications handled, 4,162, or just two-thirds, were permitted to become effective. Of the other 2,102, orders denying effectiveness were issued in only eleven cases. All the others (excepting those found not "new" and those still in process) had been found incomplete or had been withdrawn. Of the eleven orders of denial, two went to a hearing in the FDA and were affirmed; one of these led to a court proceeding, an unreported decision in which the judge made clear his unwillingness to substitute his judgment for the FDA's on an issue involving public health.[55]

In the succeeding years, though the number of applications rose, bringing the total by 1962 to about 13,000, those not permitted to become effective ranged, roughly, between 20 and 40 per cent per year; in the ten years beginning with FY 1952, only 71 per cent of 4,817 applications

49. 28 Fed. Reg. 179 (Jan. 8, 1963), adding 21 CFR §130.3.

50. 21 CFR §130.3 (d).

51. See Nelson, The New Drug Section, 6 Food Drug Cosmetic L. J. 344, 348 (1951).

52. *Id.* at 348.

53. The totals of applications filed and becoming effective, divided between drugs for human and veterinary use, are listed in the reports of the Food and Drug Administration included in the Annual Reports of the Department of Health, Education, and Welfare.

54. This occurred in FY 1962 when 411 n.d.a.'s were filed for veterinary use out of a total of 693 filings. U.S. Department of Health, Education, and Welfare, Annual Report 1962, at 341.

55. See Nelson, *supra* note 51, at 351. A lawyer familiar with the case told me of the judicial reaction. The judge's opinion is not reported.

were allowed to become effective.[56] Nevertheless, the number of hearings demanded shrank to the vanishing point. The withdrawal in 1961 of the drug Altafur was contested unsuccessfully in an administrative hearing,[57] and the year before, the suspension of diethylstilbestrol implants and injections in poultry led to a court proceeding.[58] The hearing drought continues.[59]

Problems of Communication

While the FDA was developing machinery to handle this flow of cases, the agency was wrestling with another problem which extended to all prescription drugs, new and old. The problem was how to assure communication by the manufacturer to the physician of the knowledge which the latter should have to enable him to prescribe the former's drug safely and effectively. In 1944 regulations specified ways in which the information could be made available as, for example, by a brochure or other printed matter which the label indicated either would be sent to a licensed practitioner on request or was "readily available" to him.[60]

Current regulations flatly require that "labeling on or within the package from which the drug is to be dispensed bear adequate information for its use," save only where all such information is "commonly known" to licensed practitioners.[61] Here is the legal explanation of the package insert held by the pharmacist to be dispensed to the physician who comes to him seeking knowledge. Fortunately, insert-bearing samples and the *Physicians' Desk Reference* provide him with a readier source of learning.

The package insert has, however, achieved a new role, one chiefly of importance for new prescription drugs, a role not unlike that which the

56. For the source of the data, see note 53, *supra*.
57. For a brief account of the Altafur hearing, see Mintz, The Therapeutic Nightmare 55–56 (1965).
58. Following the suspension of seven n.d.a.'s, public hearings were held between April 25 and June 17, 1960. On December 15, 1961, the Commissioner found the drugs unsafe; this order was appealed to the U.S. District Court in New Jersey. On August 20, 1964, the District Judge set aside the order (in an opinion he requested not be published) and remanded the case to the FDA for consideration pursuant to the court's order. After reconsideration, all n.d.a.'s were again ordered suspended. 30 Fed. Reg. 2315 (effective Feb. 20, 1965). See CCH, Food, Drug Cosmetic Law Rep. par. 71.551.
59. By notice in February, 1967, the FDA proposed to issue an order refusing approval of an n.d.a. for "U" series drugs of the Ubiotica Corp., the applicant having requested to file its n.d.a. over protest on the ground that the FDA had found its n.d.a. incomplete and inadequate to show the drugs' safety and effectiveness. 32 Fed. Reg. 2725. I am told that this case has not been terminated. The difficulty of fitting new drug cases into the American pattern of administrative adjudication is discussed in Cavers, Administering That Ounce of Prevention: New Drugs and Nuclear Reactors, 68 W. Va. L. Rev. 109, 233 (1966).
60. 21 CFR, 1944 Supp. 1777, §2.112.
61. 21 CFR §1.106 (b)(3)(i)(ii).

prospectus plays under the Securities Act. The content of an approved package insert represents a base line from which the FDA can measure and proceed against deviations.[62] Here is where the FDA's early identification of the prescription drug for the labeling exemption has paid unexpected dividends. This very category of drug is the one in respect to which the FDA has achieved control over advertising, filling the vacuum left when in 1938 the Wheeler-Lea Act denied the Federal Trade Comission effective control over drug advertising in medical periodicals.[63] In performing its new duties as patrolman on the Madison Avenue beat, the FDA has come to depend on the humble package insert to set limits which the creative spirits who inhabit that thoroughfare must now learn to respect.

An Attempt at Appraisal

This has been at once an overly long and an overly simplified paper. I have been able to report only a part of the story of developing drug control, and, one must remember, drug control was only a part of the FDA's total responsibilities, most of which were undergoing a comparable process of enlargement and complication. I think one might justly conclude that, considering drug control alone, this record was one of substantial accomplishment. The reader unfamiliar with the hearings of the Kefauver, Humphrey, and Fountain committees[64] and with the books that have

62. 21 CFR §1.105 ("Prescription-drug advertisements") (f)(1): "An advertisement for a prescription drug covered by a new-drug application approved after October 10, 1962 . . . shall not recommend nor suggest any use that is not in the labeling accepted in the approved new-drug application. . . . The advertisement shall present information from the approved new-drug application labeling concerning those side effects and contraindications that are pertinent with respect to uses recommended or suggested in the advertisement. . . ."

63. Federal Trade Commission Act, 15(a), 15 U.S.C. §55(a). No advertisement was to be deemed "false" if it was disseminated solely to physicians, listing quantitative ingredient information, and containing "no false representation of a material fact." Overstatement of claims can be accomplished by inference or innuendo without transgressing these conditions. Not surprisingly, reference to side effects in medical journal advertising was infrequent and sketchy. See Ruge, Regulation of Prescriptive Drug Advertising: Medical Progress and Private Enterprise, 32 Law and Contemp. Prob. 650, 657 (1967).

64. Kefauver hearings: "Administered Prices," Hearings before the Subcommittee on Antitrust and Monopoly of the Senate Judiciary Committee, 87th Cong., 1st sess. 1961, Pts. 14–26. Humphrey hearings: "Interagency Coordination in Drug Research and Regulation," Hearings before the Subcommittee on Reorganization and International Organizations of the Senate Committee on Governmental Operations, 87th Cong., 2nd sess., Pts. 1 and 2 (1962); 88th Cong., 1st sess., Pts. 3–6 (1963). Fountain hearings: "Drug Safety," Hearings before the Intergovernmental Relations Subcommittee of the House Committee on Governmental Relations, 88th Cong., 2nd sess., Pts. 1 and 2 (1964); 89th Cong., 1st sess., Pts. 3 and 4 (1965); 89th Cong., 2nd sess., Pt. 5 (1966). The Fountain hearings have been concerned chiefly with the administration of the 1962 amendments.

brought their records to public attention[65] would be surprised to find that the agency's control of drugs during the period I have been reporting was the subject of sharp attack for failure to provide adequate protection to the public.

The attack has been based mainly on particular cases where new drug applications which should have been denied or withdrawn were allowed to become, or to remain, effective. However, behind these specific mistakes are complaints that the agency did not press hard enough to secure better laws, more money, decent quarters, and abler personnel, and to achieve higher scientific standards.[66]

In evaluating the agency's record, one need not condone the failures to ask that they be set against the achievements. We do not judge a shortstop simply by counting his errors; we also ask how many chances he has accepted. On the other hand, with respect to new and prescription drugs, lives are at stake and, to return to my analogy, we are entitled to ask for something pretty close to errorless ball. Yet can one justly place the blame for creating and perpetuating conditions that make errorless ball a practical impossibility wholly upon the team—or, to revert to drug control, on the agency? Certainly no small part of the responsibility must rest on the healing professions, which were more fearful of encroachment on their preserves than insistent on improvement in the quality of the agency's work; on successive national administrations, which, until the recent past, were content to keep the FDA on low rations; on congressional watchdogs, who were willing to use the appropriation power to try to make the agency toe the line; on the industry, which exerted pressure on overloaded FDA staffs to get affirmative action rather than on the Congress to enable the agency to attract more and abler people; and, finally, on the news media, which, in the period I have covered, totally ignored the FDA between such crises as cranberries and thalidomide.

For the FDA to have carried forward the drug control program I have sketchily described with the little help it received was an achievement that I believe entitles it to a more balanced judgment than it has been accorded. However, for an agency to move from a defensive posture to one in which large-scale advances can be attempted calls for more than a display of determination on its part. Let me turn again to my baseball analogy. A ball club that has long been near the cellar may by an occasional fortunate trade move closer to the first division, but, if it is to aspire to the pennant, it needs a new manager, a lot of new players, new coaches, and a new press agent. It now seems clear that by 1962 the FDA was reaching the point where further progress required such a transformation.

65. See Harris, The Real Voice (1964); Mintz, The Therapeutic Nightmare (1965), republished with added sections commenting on developments since the original edition as By Prescription Only (1967).
66. Criticism along these lines is to be found in the hearings and books cited in notes 64 and 65, *supra*.

1938-1968: The FDA, the Drug Industry, the Medical Profession, and the Public

Louis Lasagna

The first two decades following the passage of the federal Food, Drug, and Cosmetic Act of 1938 stand in marked contrast to the decade which has just passed. Until the 1930's, the American drug industry was a pygmy. Most companies were small, and between 1932 and 1934, 3,512 firms failed, with total liabilities of $59,000,000. As late as 1939 the sales volume of Macy's department store in New York City exceeded that of any American ethical drug manufacturer. All the companies in the field could boast a total drug sales of only $301,000,000. By 1957 the figure had increased sevenfold, with the major force in the boom being the increase in ethical drugs from $149,000,000 to $1,677,000,000.

During this extraordinary period important and exciting new drugs became available to the public via the prescribing physician: the sulfonamides, penicillin, streptomycin, the antihistamines, cortisone and ACTH, the first members of the tetracycline family, chloramphenicol, and the major tranquilizers.

I believe it is true that most people—in and out of the medical profession—were not unhappy about the state of affairs at that time. The drug industry, certainly, was riding high, as were the men in the sales and advertising professions who directed drug promotion. The lag time between initial interest in a new drug and its ultimate marketing was not usually excessive, and the costs of drug development were amply repaid by the profits from sales. Doctors and their patients had available to them a large number of new drugs that could add comfort to the lives of many and were indeed at times life-saving.

Suddenly, this apparently peaceful and prosperous scene was shattered by a series of attacks—from journalists such as John Lear of the *Saturday Review*, and from the well-publicized efforts of a series of congressional groups, including the Blatnik, Kefauver, Celler, and Harris committees. The drug industry, which had come to think of itself as both successful and respected, found its officials accused of everything from overpricing to fraud. The FDA and certain clinical investigators were criticized sharply for ineptitude or dishonesty or both. The practicing physician, long accustomed to the praises of society, was portrayed as an uncritical dupe, easy prey to the blandishments of Madison Avenue.

These criticisms came from many sources—not just from congressional staff people and "muckraking" journalists, but from former FDA and pharmaceutical firm employees, academicians, and consumer groups. While each critic had his own pet complaints and orientation, certain dissatisfactions related to the quality and safety of ethical drugs were repeatedly voiced.

(1) The initial selection of drugs for clinical trial left much to be desired. Molecular relatives of already available drugs were tested even in the absence of laboratory evidence that their spectrum of activity or toxicity provided reasonable hope for advantage over marketed drugs. More important, the animal toxicity tests were highly variable from company to company, and occasionally from drug to drug within the same company. Sometimes the caliber of animal toxicity testing was shocking; furthermore, there was no legal mechanism for FDA scrutiny of preclinical data prior to human trial. Each firm was free to approach physicians on the basis of whatever appeared to the company to be adequate evidence of effectiveness and safety, and often extensive animal testing was postponed until the drug's clinical activity was assured.

(2) A good deal of clinical investigation was of poor quality. Much of the work was scientifically uninterpretable, without controls of any kind, performed by busy practitioners in their offices. Observations by these latter men were frequently limited in quantity as well as quality, so that decisions about marketing were made on the basis of pooled observations from many doctors who varied greatly in experience and competence, a technique not calculated to facilitate rational and valid decision-making by either the sponsor or the FDA medical officer monitoring the new drug application. Since such reports eventually formed much of the basis for drug advertising, it is not surprising that many promotional claims lacked substantiation when examined by critical observers.

(3) The Food and Drug Administration was forced to live in a strange Alice-in-Wonderland atmosphere, legally entitled to concern itself with the safety of a drug but not with its efficacy. This was one of the main points of concern on the part of the academic experts, who rightly considered it impossible to judge the safety of most drugs without reference to their efficacy and what they were to be used for. The FDA was thus forced to deal in a vague and paralegal way with data on efficacy and in theory could approve a drug that looked ineffective but safe. A few essentially inert drugs were in fact approved, as were inefficient drugs which harmed patients by preventing or delaying the administration of more effective agents. Many of the drugs marketed were overrated and overpromoted by their manufacturers. A scrutiny of the labeling and advertising material for drugs marketed between 1938 and 1962, for instance, reveals many examples of irrelevant material and inadequate

or absent documentation for extravagant claims. The FDA itself was held by many to be hampered by inadequate budgets, a staff deficient in both numbers and excellence, and a chaotic plan of organization. FDA officers were accused of unconscionable delays, of inexpertness in evaluating data, and of laxness both in approving drugs for sale and in removing inadequate or unsafe drugs from the market.

(4) Information on clinical drug toxicity was of low quality. The chain of reporting of a drug's untoward effects often never got started because of failure on the part of physicians to recognize or report drug reactions. Even if the chain was begun, there often proved to be weak links, with data lying buried in journals or drug house files and not brought effectively to the attention of the practicing doctor.

The hearings that terminated in the 1962 amendments were only secondarily concerned with drug efficacy and quality. Senator Kefauver's prime interest—and that of his staff—appeared to be in the area of excessive drug costs, inadequate competition, price control, and patent protection. At times, to be sure, these concerns involved the quality of drugs. For example, Kefauver's staff did evolve a set of provisions for licensing and policing drug producers as well as for guarding against the choice of generic names that were obscure and difficult to remember, so that doctors would be less reluctant to prescribe generically and thus save money for their patients and diminish the economic advantages of the larger firms.

With the aid of the thalidomide disasters, which would not have been prevented by the Kefauver-Harris Amendments, but without which the Amendments would, I am convinced, never have been passed, Congress changed the federal law on drug controls in 1962. What has been the impact of this legislation on drug development and control?

(1) The clarification of the safety-efficacy problem can hardly be interpreted as anything but desirable, at least in principle. Whether in practice the added burdens have been met by sufficient expansion of staff and improvement in processing techniques at the FDA is another matter. Some men in industry have pointed to the long delays and requests for extension of review time from FDA monitors as evidence that their gloomy predictions about what would happen have in fact been borne out, and that the public is being denied prompt access to important drugs.

(2) The requirement that the FDA be apprised of proposed human trials with new drugs has without question almost eliminated the giving of drugs to man on the basis of skimpy animal toxicity tests.[1] The complaint now is in the other direction: it is alleged by some that the tests have

1. There is little or no evidence to suggest that actual *scrutiny* by FDA monitors has prevented the clinical trial of inadequately worked-up drugs. Rather, it seems, the very *mechanism* has remedied the situation.

mushroomed out of all proportion to their worth and that some of the presently required testing, such as that for teratogenicity, is in the nature of a "we-don't-know-what-to-do-to-establish-that-a-drug-is-safe-for-the fetus-but-let's-do-something-anyway" approach.

The regulations bearing on the prompt reporting to the FDA of side effects from drugs and the mechanisms elaborated for informing the doctor of new forms of alarming toxicity have probably protected the public to a certain degree from iatrogenic disease.

(3) There has been considerable impact on the selection of drugs for clinical trial. The added costs of preclinical testing, the emphasis on the use of "expert investigators," the de-emphasis on the use of physicians in practice as "researchers," and the work and expense required to bring a drug to market have all discouraged research on "me-too" drugs. (Exciting new drugs, as in the past, do not encounter trouble in finding first-class investigators interested in working with them, despite the extra red tape now involved.)

Some of these developments, on the other hand, have probably tended to discourage imaginative, innovative research programs, which will require many millions of dollars from management over a long period of time and still may not yield a marketable drug. (Such research did not generally have high priority in the pharmaceutical industry in the past, either, but the priorities are probably even lower today.) There is a temptation in some industrial circles to look for new products abroad, in hope of buying the rights for a drug from a foreign company that has done enough clinical work to allow a good guess to be made about the compound's ultimate utility. There is also, I am sure, much less inclination on the part of industry to develop drugs needed by patients with rare diseases; such "unprofitable" research cannot be justified from the standpoint of the tough-minded economics of today's market.

(4) Despite the lack of adequate testimony on the patient consent provisions of the 1962 Amendments, the volunteer subject and patient have probably benefited—at least in regard to their personal rights—as the result of FDA and NIH regulations about human experimentation. These safeguards are embodied, in my opinion, less in the formal obtaining of informed consent than in the scrutiny, by relatively disinterested scientist peers, of protocols and consent procedures. Some research, on the other hand, has unquestionably been hampered by the new emphasis on written consent and the detailed FDA regulations interpreting and implementing the patient consent provisions.

(5) Drug advertising is now much more closely supervised by the FDA and is unquestionably less flamboyant than in the past. It may also, at the same time, be excessively restricted in some respects and more concerned with form than goals. (I shall return to this point later.)

(6) There has been a squeeze put on the small, research-minded manufacturer. The problems and costs of developing, promoting, and distributing new drugs have pushed some of these smaller firms out of the research business, or into mergers. How much of a loss this is to the public is a moot point, but it is a paradoxical result in view of the late Senator Kefauver's interests in small business.

(7) The 1962 Amendments seem not to have affected drug costs to the consumer in a dramatic way. Prices for some drugs have dropped, for a variety of reasons, including antitrust suits, but the increased costs of drug production plus the prescribing habits of doctors and the pricing habits of local pharmacists seem to have prevented any great changes in drug bills for the individual patient.

There remain some very real problems for everyone concerned with drug development and with the efficacy and safety of drugs. To begin with, the mechanism for bringing a new drug to market seems to have become excessively cumbersome and inefficient. Part of this is unquestionably a result of the requirements of the new controls, but part of the trouble seems to be simply ineptitude on the part of the various groups involved.

One has the impression, for example, that there is still too little science and too much "visceral thinking" in decisions on the part of industry and government in regard to how much preclinical testing is "enough," or what is "enough" evidence of clinical efficacy and safety.[2] The collation of data and the summarizing of clinical and preclinical reports for a new drug application (n.d.a.) has become a long, tedious business. Some useful suggestions have already been made as to how the voluminous reports could be more effectively summarized in order to expedite handling by the FDA, but one wonders how much is in fact accomplished by requiring a carload of photostated material to be assembled for the filing of an n.d.a.

One hears conflicting stories about the FDA's handling of n.d.a.'s. Some drug house employees state that they have been treated in exemplary fashion by FDA monitors; others complain of stupidity, arrogance, unreasonable demands, and delays lasting for years. The Kefauver-Harris amendments of 1962 eliminated the automatic approval of an n.d.a. by the FDA in the event that the FDA failed to respond within a period of 60 days. At present, the FDA has 6 months to review an application. Not infrequently, however, it is alleged, the sponsor fails to receive useful feedback from the FDA monitor until the 180 days are almost over and then he is told that the n.d.a. is defective in some regard, whereupon the process begins again. Or (it is said), at this point the sponsor is asked to

---

2. A special case is the requirement that Investigational New Drug forms be filed by investigators who want to employ, for diagnosis or as a research tool, time-tested chemicals such as d-xylose or lactic acid.

grant a further delay, which is almost invariably given by the sponsor, but which may last not only for months but for years.[3]

Since one rarely hears the FDA's version of this, it is difficult to know just where the truth lies. Some possible solutions do come to mind, however. To begin with, why should there not be a date set after filing for a preliminary response to the sponsor? Is not a month or two adequate time for at least a "first look" at the n.d.a. by the FDA monitor? Could he not at this time flag any obvious sources of trouble and tell the sponsor (in writing) of these? Can it really take 180 days to read and evaluate an n.d.a., or is it just that the FDA staff is overworked and no one gets to look at the application for months?

Secondly, could there not be an informal court of appeals to air disagreements between sponsors and FDA? The 1954 pesticide-chemical provisions and the 1960 color-additive provisions of the Food, Drug, and Cosmetic Act require the Secretary of HEW to establish an advisory committee of nongovernment scientists to review scientific issues whenever a qualified person requests such a review. The conclusions of these committees—whose members are chosen by the Secretary from a list suggested by the National Academy of Sciences–National Research Council—are not binding, but merely advisory. Would not such a mechanism for the FDA protect both the manufacturers and the FDA—the drug industry from inequitable bureaucracy, the FDA from unfair and irresponsible criticism? Is not some technique required which will penalize failure of the FDA to act with reasonable speed, just as the 1962 amendments were needed to avoid automatically *rewarding* the drug industry for the FDA's failure to act?

Some sort of court of appeal could also be invoked to handle those instances of alleged fraud or gross incompetence which have been considered grounds for the "black-listing" of physicians by the FDA. Such procedure is unpalatable at best—unless there are legal infractions involved which are punishable by law, in which case the law courts would seem the preferred and traditional theater of action—but at least there should be scrupulous avoidance of a "star chamber" atmosphere. It is a serious matter to impugn an investigator's honesty or competence; he should have full opportunity to know the charges against him, to face his accusers, and to offer evidence in his behalf.

There is, I believe, a need for continued upgrading of the caliber of medical personnel in the FDA, the drug industry, and academic clinical pharmacology. All three of these groups have made progress, but there is still far to go. Whereas a few decades ago it was thought shameful

3. When asked why they do not protest against unreasonable delays or demands, pharmaceutical leaders usually offer the reason that there are implicit or explicit threats of punitive or retaliatory action by the FDA if the drug houses elect to fight.

for a physician to "sell his soul" to industry, today the better drug houses are able to attract well-trained, board-certified doctors who are probably well above the average in intelligence and ability. Nevertheless, it is my impression that the general level of excellence among M.D.'s in industry is lower than that of their chemist and biologist confreres.

The FDA, too, has begun to attract better physicians, but they have further progress to make and, like the drug houses, have not as yet evolved enough imaginative ways to keep their personnel intellectually alive and high in morale. I think it vitally important for physicians in both these areas to be as highly motivated and competent as society can make them, and I doubt that this can occur without taking meaningful steps to diversify their work and to provide ways for such doctors to maintain their identities as physicians and scientists and their ties with the academic and professional community.

(It has been proposed, in a congressional bill introduced by Representative Wyatt of Oregon, that the evaluation of new drugs be turned over to the National Academy of Sciences. Without becoming involved in the pros and cons of such a move, I should like to guess that Representative Wyatt did not sound the NAS out before he introduced his bill. The Academy would not, I suspect, consider taking on this regulatory function, even if it were allowed to by the original charter.)

The universities, too, have their problems. Clinical pharmacology is on the rise in medical schools, but I have begun to doubt whether my wish, expressed some years ago, that every U.S. medical school should have a clinical pharmacology group by 1970 will be granted. Clinical pharmacology is still fighting the general decline in pharmacology as a discipline, the failure of many professors and deans to understand what clinical pharmacology is all about, the ridiculous assertion that clinical pharmacologists are "the only ones who know how to use drugs in man," or that they "know everything about everything." Clinical pharmacologists also run the danger of falling between stools, of living in limbo between departments, with neither school budgets nor the freedom to appoint young men to academic positions.

The problem of generic drugs is a most prickly one. After years of naive faith in the validity of U.S.P. standards for drug quality, it is now clear that these old-fashioned techniques are not sufficient to predict the biological performance of drugs. Both large manufacturers and small have shown their ability to make and sell drugs of inferior quality, not because of purposeful corner-cutting, but because our current quality control techniques are simply not good enough. The 1962 amendments stipulated that all batches of antibiotics be certified by the FDA, but we have all recently read of nine brands of chloramphenicol being withdrawn from the market after measurements of biological fluids in human volunteers revealed a variable and inferior performance from the generic versions of chloramphenicol.

What *are* we to demand of generic products? Better in vitro tests? In vivo measurements to show efficient absoption? How precise can we be in correlating plasma levels and therapeutic performance? How "high" is high enough for blood levels of a drug? Should plasma concentrations "peak and valley," or are "plateaus" better? Should we demand clinical trial data for every generic preparation? Can one get enough investigators to perform clinical studies on generic preparations? Is it in fact *ethical* to try an unproven generic version of an important antibiotic or drug in a seriously ill patient? Will these new requirements drive the generic manufacturer out of business? If so, what will be the impact on drug prices?

And what of the drugs marketed between 1938 and 1962? Who will restudy these? Who will undertake to show that an old analgesic mixture is superior to, and not more toxic than, its individual ingredients? Shall we take these ancient mixtures off the market, or allow them "grandfather clause" status and merely insist that their claims be toned down?

Are our consent techniques and our advertising regulations achieving the desired goals, or are we merely satisfied with making the proper gestures? Does a lengthy and detailed presentation aimed at "full disclosure" to either a volunteer subject or a doctor get across the important points, or do the small print and the excessive detail garble the message? Should information about a new drug not be more comparative in nature, placing a drug in proper perspective for the physician? The doctor not only needs to know that a new antibiotic is available, he also needs to know how it compares with those he already prescribes. In what way is the new one superior? In what way inferior? In what way safer? In what way more toxic?

This approach assumes that accurate information as to the relative merits and deficiencies of competing therapies is available, of course. But this is not the case, except in a very rough way. Clinicians sometimes act as if they are juggling cerebrally, computer-fashion, a host of probabilities for good and harm, with the final decision based on a precise balancing of the risks; this is not true, however. We must do the best that we can, of course, but there is also a need for generating data that will allow us to do better. One need only think of the abysmally poor state of our quantification of drug toxicity to appreciate how far we are from the millennium.

While thinking of research that needs doing, we might ponder the desirability of more and better research on how doctors acquire their knowledge about drugs. How much are they motivated by therapeutic potency, how much by fears of toxicity? How concerned are they with drug costs? How do we best keep doctors up to date on therapeutic matters? How can we negatively reinforce bad therapeutics, and positively reinforce exemplary therapeutics? Is the proposal for a federal compendium—one version of which sounds like a modern "five-foot-shelf" of package inserts—a realistic solution to the doctor's needs? Will such a government publication bind doctors to dosages, indications, etc., that hamper the practice of good medicine?

And what of the public? Is it really desirable for the patient to remain a relatively ignorant consumer, unable to function effectively as a force for quality prescribing? If not, how do we best educate the public? We know that some patients fail to fill their prescriptions, and many more fail to take medicines as prescribed. How do we modify this behavior? The consumer is often said to be interested, quite reasonably, in drug costs. Does he know about the studies that have been done on prescription costs? Is he aware of the contribution made by the pharmacist's pricing practices to drug costs? Does he realize that prescribing generically is no guarantee of a lower drug bill? Does he know that the way he dresses and the color of his skin can affect the price of his prescription?

While on the subject of economics, I cannot resist voicing some anxiety about the possibly deleterious effect on industrial research of a decline in revenues. The ethical drug houses of this country have not had much fiscal reason to complain in the past. Their stockholders have fared well. The drug industry has probably suffered, in fact, from the relative ease with which money could be made from drugs. As with the too-ready availability of NIH research funds, such a situation encouraged—or at least tolerated—the second-rater. The penalties for mediocrity were neither dramatic nor inevitable. I believe this situation no longer obtains. I suspect that drug houses are in for some leaner years—not for famine, but for less fat. This may be to the good, but I have already hinted at the possibility that long-range commitments to research, especially for "gamble-type" research, may be decreasing, in a preoccupation with short-term profit statements.

If this does occur, what should society do? Should we think of special tax credits or other incentives? Should the NIH undertake large-scale support of drug development if enthusiasm could be mustered for drug searches in the nonindustrial world? I would be happier if we could at least count on a continuing appraisal of this situation over the next decade. It would require confidential surveys, and candor and honesty on the part of the researchers and management people in industry, and it would not be an easy task, but I believe that it would serve the public well to monitor this particular pulse.

Commentary

Vincent A. Kleinfeld

There is one lesson which every lawyer in the food and drug area knows: it is a sad fact of life that the food and drug area is what lawyers call *sui generis*, in a class by itself. For example, an attorney in any other field of law usually follows a certain procedure when his client asks a question: may the client legally do this or may he not? The lawyer reads the law, scrutinizes the legislative history, analyzes the problems, and peruses the judicial decisions, and then he often can say to his client, "Yes, you may do this," or, "No, you may not do this." The unfortunate lawyer in the food and drug area has to do this, but then he continues. He has resolved the problem to his legal satisfaction; clearly, in his opinion, as a conservative lawyer, it is fine, you may do this. But now he scratches his head: "What will the Food and Drug Administration say?" This is an entirely different problem. This is no criticism; it is, again I say, a fact of life. The Food and Drug Administration may well take a position predicated on its desire to construe the law in order to give the consumer the greatest possible protection, whether or not Congress had this in mind. So he must think about that.

He must also think about the fact, perhaps a good one, that the courts in this area of the law tend to equate the Food and Drug Administration with God, motherhood, and country. This is also a fact of life. He must also know that it is very expensive to fight—these damn lawyers need a lot of money! And there is this devastating publicity which somehow gets to Drew Pearson and Morton Mintz and congressional committees! This, also, the lawyer in this field knows. Now it may well be, unfortunately, that many drug manufacturers and distributors have not realized this yet, but they had better do so. The average man is certainly an amateur in many fields, but in the fields of food and drugs he is a decided amateur; we cannot sell drugs as if they were shoes and ships and sealing wax—they are too important. Part of the continued evolution and revolution in the drug industry is caused, I think, by the failure of many companies to get it into their thick heads that drugs are too important to be handled like any other commodity.

Let us turn to what has been discussed above: what do we need in the way of regulatory legislation? It is a tough problem from the viewpoint of the lawyer, the scientist, and the public. If our sole aim is to give the public the greatest possible protection, there is an infinite number of laws and regulations that can be passed and promulgated. That is a wonderful end, and perhaps we must continue to pass more and more extensive laws. I am not saying this is good or bad. Perhaps the answer in enveloped in one's personal philosophy and in one's ideas of the philosophy of government. Let us see what further can be done, and perhaps may be done in the future, in respect to regulation of the drug industry. Time passes and all sorts of things change. The 1906 Food and Drug Act could not have been passed in 1848, the 1938 act could not have been passed in 1906, the Drug Amendments of 1962 could not have been passed in 1938, and only the good Lord knows what is going to be passed in the future.

Let us see what more can be done by a zealous Food and Drug Administration, a zealous congressional committee, and a Congress that wants to aim at this wonderful end of giving the public the greatest possible protection in the field of drugs. Perhaps we should license every drug manufacturer; this will presumably come to pass. Perhaps every piece of advertising and labeling should have to be cleared to the satisfaction of the Food and Drug Administration before it is utilized. Certainly this will cut down on false and misleading claims, or on the failure to give a proper brief summary in an advertisement, or adequate full disclosure in a label. Perhaps we should have an inspector in every drug plant; we have one in every meat plant. Perhaps every batch of every Rx drug should have to be certified by the Food and Drug Administration. All these things would undoubtedly give greater protection to the consumer. Since there have been instances where a company, or some officials—even scientists—have done things they should not, perhaps all testing should be performed by a government agency. Perhaps we should nationalize the drug industry. I suppose then we would not have these problems about fraud, false and misleading claims, failure to give full disclosure of side effects, contraindications, and so on. And this may be inevitable; it may be that that is what this country wants.

I suppose in each instance the doctor and the Food and Drug Administration, before either using or approving a drug, must weigh how good it is, how serious is the condition for which it is offered, and what are the side effects. If Congress wants to increase this area of protection, as I am sure it will, it also must weigh (and I suppose will weigh) against the greater protection that the consumer will undoubtedly have, the increased cost, the increase in personnel in whichever agency or agencies are chosen to perform these tasks, and the lengthy and inevitable delays. Then Congress will have to decide whether each particular step forward in increasing the protection of the consumer is so important that it will outweigh the countervailing considerations. I think the problem is an extremely complicated one, and perhaps, as I have stated, the answer lies in one's philosophy of government as to whether, even in as vital a field as foods and drugs, we want to put the state so comprehensively into the area. Certainly we know that it is not only in this country—or in the last fifty years—that the state has felt compelled to protect the consumer. There was a provision on weights and measures in the Magna Carta, and we know that there was a prohibition against the eating of pork in Leviticus. We can go back as far as we want in recorded history to realize that this is a perennial problem. In the Middle Ages in England, for example, it was found that there were earnest entrepreneurs who were using clay in flour and water in beer and ale. This underlying quality of greed, I am afraid, has been with us for a long time.

Dr. Lasagna has pointed out that under the original new-drug section of the law as passed in 1938 the only criterion was safety. The problem of effectiveness was met in a large measure under the 1938 act, however, before the 1962 amendments. It was clear that the only criterion in the new-drug section was safety, but it was not long before the Food and Drug Administration took the position, and properly so, that if a drug was offered for a serious condition and was ineffective for it, the drug was not safe. That took care of the biggest problem on effectiveness, the problem occasioned by drugs offered for serious conditions. If it was not offered for a serious condition, the Food and Drug Administration would often say, in approving a new drug application, "We are approving your new drug application because we have to, since we cannot say it is unsafe, but your claims are on your responsibility"; or, "We have to approve your new drug application, but if you put your drug on the market, we will seize it next week, and maybe we will prosecute you." All these things were covered and contained in the original 1938 act.

Actually, a number of things that were done in the 1962 amendments could have been accomplished by the then existing 1938 act. The FDA had required full disclosure in labeling prior to 1962, and regulations could have been issued long before 1962 making serious changes in the investigational new drug procedures—the government had the authority. Of course, in that instance and in other instances, if it had done so, there would have been tremendous screams from industry, but the FDA has not been bothered too much in the past by these screams. I think the bigger problem, which has been pointed out, was that there were not enough funds to do it; the power was there, even before the 1962 amendments. The 1938 act was a very strong law; its biggest weakness was the fact that it did not directly control the advertising of prescription drugs.

Another point made by Dr. Lasagna is that the recent increases in FDA's regulations have pushed some of the smaller drug firms out of the research business. This undoubtedly is true, and it certainly has pushed and probably will push many small drug firms and generic manufacturers out of business. Senator Kefauver's staff, I think, was horrified to realize that this was again another fact of life. The increasing regulations and the increasing regulatory activity, which I think are necessary, cost a lot of money. So again we have different policy considerations. I suppose most of us think it is healthy to keep small businesses around. On the other hand, we have a counterbalancing policy consideration, which I think is more important. We want to give the consumer the greatest possible protection, and we have to have, for example, tough regulations for good manufacturing practices.

Now, let us say somebody wants to get a new drug application approved. The big company may be brave enough, and have enough funds, and have the requisite talent, for it, from time to time, to reach its own conclusion that a product it wishes to market is not a new drug because it is, in fact, generally recognized as safe and effective by experts. The small manufacturer does not have access to that talent, to that expertise, necessary to reach the judgment. All he can do is ask what really amounts to a rhetorical question of the Food and Drug Administration. He can do that terrible thing, writing a letter to the government, and he can say, "Is my product, with its formulation and labeling, a new drug?" Well, this is, in 95 per cent of the times, a rhetorical question; the answer, of course, is "Yes." Sometime even a bigger company uses what I call the conduit approach: "I have a problem: is my product a new drug, is my advertising or labeling okay, am I giving full disclosure or an adequate brief summary, are my representations sound?" Let me give you a deep secret—when a piece of paper is put in front of a government official, there is an immediate reflex action, a knee-jerk reaction, he reaches for a pencil! If you talk informally with a Food and Drug Administration official, he will tell you, "There are instances when somebody asks me a question and I say to myself, 'why did the damn fool ask me the question? I have to give him the answer he does not want.'" Thus, if a small generic manufacturer uses this conduit approach, and he probably has to, he will never get into trouble with the government, but, more often than not, he will not be able to do a lot of things that his big competitors can do. I do not know the answer. It is just a very interesting fact and it is a tough fact of life. Maybe it has to be that way.

Let us talk about new drug applications. We have all heard about new drug applications and delays. Perhaps we can have committees set up by, let us say, the National Academy of Sciences–National Research Council, not to make the final decision—by no means. But it probably would be helpful to both the drug industry and the Food and Drug Administration to provide for the setting up of such a committee at the request of either the drug firm involved or the Food and Drug Administration. Such a procedure exists with respect to other sections of the law. I think it would be very helpful here. I am afraid that occasionally you will find a doctor in an agency who, to use an old government expression, "wants to keep his nose clean." If he says "no," he is in good shape. No congressional committee is ever going to criticize him for having approved a new drug application, since, if the drug is never marketed, there cannot, I assume, be any side reactions. So, there is the unfortunate tendency in some to say "no"; to remember thalidomide; to remember that somebody got a medal for saying "no." Nobody, no zealous congressman or committee, perhaps acting fairly, perhaps, however, looking for a little publicity, can ever put him on the stand and say, "Why did you approve this?"

I think we know, I believe I am right, that a drug can be marketed after a tremendous amount of exploration and testing on rats and mice and monkeys and elephants and perhaps thousands of human guinea pigs and everything is fine. Then it is put out on the market, is used by a million people, and 0.01 per cent get a blood problem and perhaps die. Now the doctor who did an honest job in approving the new drug application may be hailed up before a committee, or at least the agency may be hailed up, and asked "Why did you approve this?" It is relatively simple to look back and criticize, particularly if one is looking for publicity. Setting up a committee of learned scientists in the National Research Council may stiffen the back of some official who, unfortunately, may unconsciously be saying "no" or sending "incomplete" letter after "incomplete" letter just one day before the statutory 180 days have elapsed, because this way he just will not get into trouble.

Some of the speakers mentioned these "incomplete" letters, which I fondly call the "incomplete gimmick." There may have been some reason for it in the dark, pre-thalidomide, pre-Kefauver, and pre-Goddard days, because there was a provision in the 1938 act, a bad one, that a new drug application would automatically be made effective, really approved, if the government did not act within the statutory period of time; everybody says 60 days, but actually it could have been 180 days. I believe that it does not make sense, under any circumstances, for a new drug application to be approved when it has not been scrutinized by the FDA. One of the changes made in the 1962 amendments was to remove the provision for an n.d.a. becoming automatically effective if the statutory time passed without action by the FDA. This was changed by the 1962 amendments, and everybody fondly hoped—expected—that there was no longer any sound reason for the "incomplete" gimmick, but it did not come to pass and the ploy is still used. This raises a problem, because when an n.d.a. comes in to an FDA official, he may put it in the bottom of the file, and wait 179 days, and then write a letter saying your n.d.a.

is incomplete for 1, 2, or 52 reasons. And when an attempt is made to meet these reasons by a further submission, the 180 days start running anew—and do not ever send in a revised piece of labeling or change a semicolon because that period is going to start running all over again, and you may get any number of "incomplete" letters. I think this should be met in some fashion: not, certainly, by reverting to the very bad provision of automatic effectiveness, but perhaps by requiring a report to Congress, or to the President perhaps, of what has happened in the past year in connection with new drug applications—who did what to whom, how long it took, and why. I am a firm believer in checks and balances, and I think some check, some balance, is needed in this area.

One point raised by Dr. Lasagna is, I think, extremely important. No matter what good legislation we may have, I think every lawyer engaged in administrative law knows that what is equally important, or probably more important, is the quality of the administrative agency. The FDA has always been one of my favorite agencies. But whereas there used to be two doctors in the new drug division, there are dozens now. It is vital, I think, to get into the Food and Drug Administration numbers of physicians who are dedicated and highly qualified. There are many there now; we need more. First of all, you have to pay them well; it takes an awfully long time before a doctor makes any money anyway. He can go out in private practice eventually and do very well. He is a human being with the frailties that we all have. To get him into the government and to keep him you have to pay him adequately, and you have to give him tenure. You have to back him up when he needs backing up, even against Drew Pearson or some congressional committee. We must do another thing, it seems to me, and I remember mentioning this to former Commissioner Dunbar way back in the dark old days. The kind of man you want and need desperately is probably not going to be satisfied sitting behind a desk day after day, year after year, reading five-foot shelves of new drug applications. He has got to be permitted, in fact required, to do something else. Let him go to the Public Health Service for a while, make him go to the hospitals and accompany somebody on rounds, get him away from that desk, or otherwise something is going to happen to him. I remember that when I was in the government—the halcyon days—I used to say that there ought to be a law passed immediately that every government employee, including myself, should be compelled to change his job every five years; otherwise, one's horizons necessarily become narrowed, limited. If you want to get the best men into government—and we need them desperately, particularly in the fields of medicine and pharmacology—we have got to pay them well, we have got to make their work more interesting; I believe that is the most important thing we can say today.

Commentary

Wallace F. Janssen

June 25, 1968, marked the thirtieth anniversary of the present federal Food, Drug, and Cosmetic Act. That law, like the Act of 1906, started out as a primarily punitive statute to protect consumers through actions in the courts, but it contained significant authority to prevent violations through regulatory procedures. A series of major amendments extended the application of this principle of preventive enforcement, beginning with the insulin amendment in 1941, followed by penicillin certification in 1945, pesticide tolerances in 1954, food additives in 1958, color additives in 1960, and drug effectiveness in 1962. The general pattern of all these controls is significant: industry and government work at the same job, each being given specific duties. Industry must submit scientific data on safety and effectiveness, proposed labeling, and samples for testing. Government is to evaluate the evidence presented and make certain decisions: to certify or not to certify a batch, to set a tolerance, to approve or not to approve the marketing of a drug. This pattern of shared responsibility requires communication and understanding to make it work. It cannot work without the capability of carrying on scientific research and testing procedures, again a matter of joint interest by government and industry. Advancing technology, evidenced by the drug revolution to which Mr. Cavers has referred, is the underlying force, stimulating both the progress of the law and the further progress of science. More than ever, the law is an instrument of change, tending to promote rational therapeutics, to insure reliable therapeutic products, and to convey the information needed to use them properly. Dr. Lasagna's numerous, deeply probing questions have indicated the complications involved in reaching these objectives.

Where is the dividing line between history and news? The record before us is of course incomplete. Future readers of this record no doubt will find it helpful to consult the most recent annual reports and speeches in order to get up to date on the topics we are discussing. In May, 1968, Commissioner Goddard, in a speech to the American Pharmaceutical Association, reported the progress made in the mass review of drug effectiveness which has been carried on by the Drug Research Board of the National Academy of Sciences–National Research Council. Over

3,600 drug formulations were involved, with perhaps 5 "me-too" variants
for each. These were the drugs cleared for safety but not effectiveness in
the period from 1938 to 1962. It must be the largest program in history
to evaluate the validity of therapeutic claims. In January the Academy's
first judgments, involving 4 drugs, were published in the *Federal Register*.
Today—May, 1968—some 200 are awaiting publication.

Dr. Goddard also reported on the elimination of the backlog of
pending new drug applications, which at one point in 1966 totaled around
300. "President Johnson asked me to do something about the situation,"
said Dr. Goddard. "We promised to him that FDA would eliminate the
backlog by July 1, 1967."

Dr. Goddard then recounted the steps taken to meet this deadline.
"Today," he said, "we stay fairly current. That is, on some days we have
several n.d.a.'s pending beyond the 180-day limit. But we manage to
catch up. We are, of course, tougher on drug sponsors. It seems sensible
and in the public interest that we give our attention to those submittals
that have been professionally prepared. They reveal a sponsor with a
sense of good management. For those who still send in poorly prepared
materials, we have a simple mechanism: we send it back—in some instances, with prejudice." In this connection, a substantial improvement
in the quality of applications has been noted since 1967.

A very great increase in use of product recall as a means of insuring
safe and effective drugs should be mentioned. In the fiscal year 1967 drug
recalls increased 45 per cent, from 446 to 651. If a recall will provide
better protection to the public than a seizure, the current FDA policy is
to urge a recall.

Most of the provisions of the 1962 drug amendments have been discussed by the contributors, but the record of this meeting would be
incomplete if I did not mention two which have an important bearing on
drug control. These are the authority to establish the Good Manufacturing
Practice Regulations for drug plants, and the requirement that all drug
establishments be registered by the Food and Drug Administration.

All three papers in this section refer to efforts to establish and maintain *drug standards*, starting with the first federal law, the Import Drugs
Act of 1848. Very significant was the inauguration of the Contact Committees of the two drug manufacturing groups which became the present
Pharmaceutical Manufacturers' Association. The history of analytical
methods for drug control is very much a part of the history of drug regulation and is basic to the legislative history. Without the methods, regulatory
laws would be unworkable. Here is a field for further development from
the historical standpoint.

Again we are up against what my friend Professor Young likes to call
the "cutting edge" of history. Today, again, we are confronted with the

realization that the drug supply includes too many products that do not meet the ever more demanding standards of excellence that must be required of drugs. It is a serious situation, made more pressing by the public interest in the so-called generic drug issue. Do all drugs really work as promised by their sponsors ? Are they therapeutically equivalent if they are chemically—or generically—equivalent ? How good, really, is our drug supply ? Hence the significance of a new FDA approach through establishment of a National Center for Drug Analysis in the quarters of its former St. Louis District—quarters, I may say, which are far from adequate. Here methods are being developed for analyzing drug samples on a mass production basis with automated equipment. And this, necessarily, is only a beginning on the complex of difficult problems that Dr. Lasagna has dealt with.

Concerning the informal "court of appeals" idea which he has mentioned, the FDA seems to be moving in that direction through the numerous medical advisory committees, both standing and *ad hoc*, which have been created in various areas.

Speaking of courts, little attention has been given to the fundamental importance of the fact that the federal Food, Drug, and Cosmetic Act is a law with teeth. Experience continues to demonstrate that prosecutions, seizures, and injunctions, with their collateral effects in the areas of publicity and civil liability, are both the greatest deterrents to violations and the greatest incentive to good practices. Great damage is done to consumer protection when it gets around that prosecution is unlikely. Even the ethical drug manufacturer can be tempted by the pressure to reduce costs and be competitive, with the result that control is neglected. The dishonest and the quacks, who are always present, respect only the strong arm of law enforcement.

A basic theme inherent and explicit in all the papers is the medical communication problem. As Dr. Lasagna has put it: "How do we best keep doctors up to date on therapeutic matters ? *How can we negatively reinforce bad therapeutics, and positively reinforce exemplary therapeutics ?*" This, indeed, comes close to summarizing the import of all that has been said here about drug control.

Discussion

Dr. Dowling: The last speaker has noted that certain trends have run through all these papers. One trend, certainly, was evolution. The papers have discussed, or at least touched upon, the evolution of many things. I would like to ask about the possibility of evolution not only up to now but also into the future in two areas.

One of these areas has to do with what our attorneys said about decisions in the courts being made poorly. Many speakers have stated that advisory committees are being set up. I happen to have pushed for such committees and to have been on a number of them, but it seems to me that an advisory committee is only one step. The committee is supposed to include experts, but generally the other side is not heard; such a committee tends to be composed of people who have a certain attitude and have expressed it already. For instance, the last one that I was on had to do with chloramphenicol. As I look back on that meeting, there was no one there who really felt that chloramphenicol should be used almost *ad lib.*, and yet I believe some doctors feel this way. I think such persons should be heard—this is my point. The next step, then, seems to me to be a committee in which the industry participates, a committee which they request to look into something and which hears the opinions of persons with differing viewpoints. I can see a disadvantage, in that, if there are very many of these committees, if a committee is requested every time a decision comes up, it will really bog down the work of the Food and Drug Administration. I would like to know whether the lawyers think this is likely to happen.

A further step, it seems to me—here I am way out in quicksand—and a step that does not relate only to the Food and Drug Administration but also to other scientific areas in the government, is this: If we have groups of lawyers who after a lifetime of work in the law are considered to be prominent and proficient in their profession, and able to rise above petty attitudes, and who therefore are appointed to the higher state courts, the federal courts, and finally the Supreme Court, why should we not look toward courts of scientists to do exactly the same thing with regard to scientific decisions?

The other area of evolution is one which has come through clearly. Our emotions tell us that we want to do everything we can to improve the whole situation with regard to drugs. Actually, what we are able to do at any particular time depends upon technology. As chemistry and micro-biology evolved, it became possible to do something about the purity, identity, and quality of drugs, and these were the first things that were taken care of. Because of a strong emotional reaction, people also wanted to do something about poisons. They also worked early on quack remedies and did a great deal, at least in the advertising area. The labeling and advertising of prescription drugs were tackled only later, presumably because they were harder to get at. It was obvious that the blatant claims of the quacks were wrong, but it was very difficult to make a case in court, or so I would assume, that the slight nuances found in some of the advertisements for prescription drugs were misleading. People worked on adverse effects and efficacy early, but did not really have the tools. At first, crude attempts were made to test the efficacy, and to a certain extent the adverse effects, on humans. It is one of my pet theses that when a person tries a drug himself, the experiment is often done poorly and without real objective scientific criteria. Testing on humans was discarded to a large extent, because the laboratory people had developed animal techniques, often for other reasons, which could be utilized for the study of drugs. Then we got into a bind five or ten years ago when we were relying on animal techniques and were not even studying a drug in humans until it went out on the market. We have caught up with ourselves now with the 1962 act.

Mr. Cavers: Dr. Dowling has been referring to a problem that I think, from the standpoint of the lawyer looking at this field or even of the scholar looking at it, is one of the most challenging and fascinating problems that exists in the area, and that is the possibility of using advisory boards or some form of mechanism, whether advisory or decision-making, in which the applicant for a new drug, or the opponent of the withdrawal of a drug, can get a hearing in which he feels greater confidence than the hearing before the agency that has been pursuing him or denying him what he wants. I do not, thus far, feel that we have resolved this problem. We do have statutory provision for advisory boards in the pesticides field and, I believe, in color additives, when the product may be at issue. My belief is that the advisory board for pesticides is very seldom used. Perhaps Mr. Janssen can tell us on how many occasions we have had to use advisory boards on pesticides.

Mr. Janssen: If you were to consider the number of committees vis-à-vis the number of tolerances set, I suppose it would be small. On the other hand, we have had quite a few. I could not give you a number, but I would say that a committee is requested quite frequently.

Mr. Cavers: Apparently it has never gone beyond the committee stage into litigation.

One of the problems we have had is that, for this kind of decision-making, the law has relied very much on the adversary process. By and large I think the scientific fraternity abhors the adversary process, and it also can be in this area a very expensive process in terms of the time required for each side to mobilize its views. Whether we can adapt the mechanism of the hearing board to meet the special needs of this field, I am not sure. I worked on a staff study for the Joint Committee on Atomic Energy, out of which we produced a special design for a hearing board to pass on the applications for the construction of power reactors. Ultimately we wound up with the development of a panel from which, for each case, two or three technically qualified persons are chosen to serve with a presiding officer who is trained in presiding over administrative proceedings—which is a circumlocution for saying "a lawyer." These boards have been functioning, although they have been complained of at times as time-consuming. They have not run into the problem of adversary proceedings very often because, as a rule, in these situations there is no contest. Nonetheless, these are public hearings. I think the area is one that deserves study, and I think it is a study in which the legal profession and the medical and pharmaceutical professions can very usefully join with persons with experience in administration.

Mr. Kleinfeld: I think there is much in what Dr. Dowling says, though I do not know how to meet it exactly. First of all, I must repeat that it is no use going to court whether you are right or wrong. If the Food and Drug Administration yells "hazard" or "danger," you are not going to get one judge out of a hundred to hold against the Food and Drug Administration; this I can testify to from very bitter experience since I have been in private practice and with the government. When you are before a judge, it makes practically no difference whether the government is right or wrong. The government attorney looks up gravely at the judge and says, "Your Honor, the Food and Drug Administration . . ."—there is a pause right there—"takes the position that this product is dangerous; it may cause death either directly or because it keeps the patient away from the knife, the X-ray machine, radium. If Your Honor wishes to take the grave responsibility of substituting your judgment for that of the Food and Drug Administration . . ."—another pause. That is it, and perhaps rightly: the judge is not qualified in this area.

What are we going to do? I think setting up committees is a very good thing for the reason I mentioned, and I do not think it would cause any undue delays; I do not know how there could be any more undue delays than we have now, anyway. I think it would work. It would help the FDA. Also, if we did go to a court sometime when we really felt the FDA was wrong, and we had a report from the committee which differed from the Food and Drug Administration, maybe the court would try to do a fair, honest, and impartial job.

Another possibility which I have never seen discussed is this. I do not want scientists to be judges; I do not think they are fit for it. Also, anybody who has been in litigation knows that a good lawyer, by the time he is through a particular case, may know as much as the learned expert on the stand. We have a Court of Tax Appeals to which one can go with respect to a tax decision made by the Internal Revenue Service. We might have a Court of Food and Drug Appeals, so that these judges— if not immediately, then after a passage of time—would get the expertise and self-confidence to reach decisions that would be sound legally and scientifically.

Dr. Whittet: In Britain, we have made provision in the new medicines legislation for committees under the new Medicines Commission, and we have also stipulated that no drug will be turned down without one of these appropriate committees being considered. We regard this as a safeguard for the manufacturers. The committees will not be asked to see everything; it may be only a very occasional instance where this will be done.

I should like to refer to two other items which previous speakers have mentioned. One was the possibility of registration of all drug firms. Although we in Britain are not yet in the Common Market, we are in the Council of Europe, which is the six Common Market countries plus Britain and Switzerland, and we are also in the European Free Trade Association, which contains about eight countries. Of those, we are the only one which does not have registration of new drugs at the moment —we have the voluntary Committee on Safety of Drugs (Dunlop Committee) procedure—but we shall be having registration. Eventually we hope to get reciprocal recognition of registration to save firms from having to apply to a dozen countries or more or at least to enable them to put the application in exactly the same form to each country.

The other item was the reference by two people to good manufacturing practice. This is very much in the public mind in pharmaceutical circles in Europe at the moment. You probably know that WHO has put out a tentative scheme for it. The European Free Trade Association— EFTA—and the Council of Europe are also studying this, and I hope that something reasonably uniform will come out of it. Obviously it would be best if WHO could do it, but considering that WHO has 120 members, from advanced countries like the United States down to newly formed nations, it is probably impossible. But I think it may well be possible with small groups like EFTA and the Council of Europe. That would be a start and other countries could come in later.

Dr. Lasagna: The fascinating thing that keeps cropping up, it seems to me, is how the evolution of controls at a given point in history lulls society into a state of relative contentment which, in retrospect, seems not at all justified. For example, listening to discussions of controls on the purity of some of the ancient "medicaments" which now are considered quite inert conjures up the image of controls on the purity, melting point, and shelf-life of a ghost. We finally get to the *USP* type of controls and standards, which lull us into the belief that drugs meeting those standards are performing well, and then we find out that the standards are not adequate. Nowadays, we are being lulled again into a false sense of security by focusing on regulatory measures aimed at what is referred to as "maximal protection of the public." Too often this is translated into protection either for the pocket or for the body against the toxic effects of drugs. I submit that in fact we ought to be worrying about the maximal *health* of the public, which involves a happy environment for the efficient elaboration of the new drugs so desperately needed to treat some of the things that we cannot treat now. It is very hard to quantify the harm to the public of not having these drugs, or to dramatize such a lack, yet it is the other side of the coin. It is easier to see how legislation and regulations hinder the development of new remedies than how they might help. I sense a lack of appreciation in public discussions for that aspect of regulatory activity.

Dr. Dowling: This last point of Dr. Lasagna's is extremely important. There is one analogy which may be relevant. In the Division of Biologics Standards at the National Institutes of Health, which regulates, as you know, vaccines and serums, they have a research group and are fostering research in the area they are regulating. The Food and Drug Administration has never done this, except for limited research in methodologies. If we could really make the FDA into a research entity as well as a regulatory entity, we could have this attitude. I personally do not see any harm in it.

Mr. Cowen: I would like to direct a question to Mr. Kleinfeld. Am I correct in my memory that prior to or during the early part of the Kefauver hearings the relationships between the committee and the FDA were strained?

Mr. Kleinfeld: Certainly it is my understanding that they were quite strained, but I think you perhaps might direct that to Mr. Janssen. I have never been with FDA. Mr. Janssen, however, is.

Mr. Cowen: I wonder if that could be explained. What was there in the early part of the hearings that made the FDA and the Kefauver committee almost at odds for a while?

Mr. Janssen: The story of what happened to the FDA in the years since around 1958 is very complicated, and no one has really told it yet. I have read some books based on the hearings, but none of them tells the whole story. The hearings were very extensive but they did not always give the FDA viewpoints.*

Dr. Young: I would really like to second what Mr. Janssen said. One point, however, that I think was of extreme importance in the suspicion that fell upon the Food and Drug Administration and that helped strain the relationships between the Kefauver committee and the FDA was the revelation that one high FDA official had taken in a quarter million dollars over seven years in payments from certain journals in his particular field. I do not doubt at all that this case was one of the factors, but I also do not doubt that there were a number of others.

Dr. Lasagna: At least part of the trouble arose, as I remember it, from the fact that there were several FDA employee malcontents who had free access to the Kefauver committee's ears and who were highly critical of some of the things going on in the FDA. They were equally critical of the drug industry, but they were very critical of some of their superiors. I do not know what all the other reasons may have been, but I am sure that was one source of trouble between the FDA and the committee.

Dr. Dowling: To follow that up, I wonder if you did not have this polarization because the Food and Drug Administration, as one of the contributors pointed out, had been very conservative over a number of years, partly because the administration was conservative and partly because they had always been in the habit of asking, and were very proud of the fact that they were asking, for low appropriations. One of the officials actually told me this years ago, that the FDA did not go in and ask for big sums and that the Congress thought highly of them because of this. Their appropriations were low, abysmally low. Commissioner Larrick was trying to move out of this position as best he could, and I believe he called the first Citizens' Advisory Committee for this reason, among others. He was hoping that increased appropriations would be one of the effects, and they turned out to be.

You had, then, a very conservative administration which did not implement fully the steps which, at least so Mr. Kleinfeld said, it could have taken under existing law in relation to efficacy and some other things. It did not relate very much to the scientific community, either. On the other hand, there were those whom Dr. Lasagna called malcontents—other people call them "Young Turks"—that is, people who wanted to get something done in a hurry. Because these groups were so far apart, it was possible to drive a wedge—a characteristic, shall we say, of congressional committees—in order to get their message across. If you have a more progressive Food and Drug Administration, then the Young Turks

---

* When they become available, the FDA papers in the Johnson Library at Austin, Texas, are expected to provide a major source concerning the period.

in it—and let's hope there will always be Young Turks in every organization—will not be so far away from the administration that they feel they
cannot relate to it and so have to go somewhere else.

Mr. Janssen: Dr. Dowling used the word "evolution" a while ago, and I
think this is very important. The balance between technology and regulation is constantly being upset by the progress of technology. Regulation
becomes obsolete continuously and society must try to solve the problems
a new way. This, I think, has a good deal to do with the underlying
motivation.

Dr. Young: One other theme that would be worth focusing on, though it
has come out in one aspect and another in the discussions, is the relationship between the regulated and the regulators at any given moment in
history, particularly with reference to the prevailing political climate of
the executive branch and of the Congress. I alluded to the situation in the
1920's, when the regulated and the regulators were close to each other,
but in such a way that, because of the flavor of the administration, the
business groups had almost an upper hand. A little later on with the New
Deal this was to shift. In the 1950's it was to shift again in the other direction, but now there is agitation for even more reform. Nevertheless, the
Food and Drug Administration and regulated industries are having
meaningful conversation, it seems to me, in some areas. There is discussion
with regard to handling of food problems through self-certification.
There is discussion that may lead to a better situation without a new law,
or perhaps without such a drastic law, in connection with cosmetics. Not
too long ago a confrontation with some experts present had at least some
success in connection with regulations on the handling of aspirin for
children and probably made a law unnecessary at that moment. All the
kinds of pressures in the background from the Congress and the President,
and the varying relationships between the business community, the Congress, and the President, give to the problems of drug control an ever
changing and always intriguing environment.

Dr. Blake: The hour grows late. As Chairman, I must reluctantly exercise
my prerogative to call this meeting to a halt. Before I do so, let me express,
on behalf of the National Library of Medicine and the Josiah Macy, Jr.
Foundation, our thanks to the contributors and to all of you who have
participated in these informative and stimulating papers and discussions.

Index

Academy of Medicine, Paris: Commission on Secret and New Remedies, 7
Accum, Fredrick, 18–19
Adulteration Acts, nineteenth-century Great Britain: exclusion of drugs from, 20, 22; execution of, 22–25
Adulteration of drugs: *British Pharmacopoeia* in control of, 16–26; definition of, 15, 24; nineteenth-century France, legal measures against, 9; nineteenth-century Great Britain, 19–20
—detection by microscopy: 16–17; optical techniques, 17; organoleptic means, 16–17
—legislation against: adoption of state laws, 107; influence of American Pharmaceutical Association, 106–7; influence of *Pharmacopoeia of the United States*, 107; responsibility shifted from pharmacist to suppliers, 107
Agriculture, Department of: 127–28; *see* Chemistry, Bureau of Alchemy, 52, 54
Alexandrian medicine: use of bleeding and drugs, 52
Alkaloids: discovery of, 10
—vegetable: industry taking over pharmacy production of, 73–74
American Institute of Homeopathy: disagreement with AMA over proprietary drugs, 121
American Journal of Pharmacy, 99–100
American Medical Association: and federal drug regulation, 120, 127–31; changes in policy, commentary on, 132–34; contributed to *Pharmacopoeia of the United States*, 120; early twentieth century, therapeutic nihilism in, 112–13; educational crusade to eliminate proprietary medications, 117–19; hostility toward compulsory health insurance, 129; mentioned, 118, 121, 122, 148; published *New and Nonofficial Remedies*, 114; revealed defects in federal and state drug laws, 115–17; *see also* Council on Pharmacy and Chemistry; Seal of Acceptance program

American Pharmaceutical Association: attempts to control drug quality, 100, 105–7; mentioned, 113, 118
Ampoule, 77
Analgesics: appraisal of, 59–70; barbiturates as, central nervous system reaction to, 59
Anesthetics, 59
Animal experimentation, in evaluation of drugs: seventeenth century, 55; eighteenth century, 56; mentioned, 190; pain studies, 62, 69
Antitrust Laws in 1938, 129
Apothecaries, Paris: organized into College of Pharmacy in 1777, 3
Apothecary-physician relationship: influence on drug control, 46
Apothecary shops, Paris: inspection of, 3
Arsphenamine: discovery as antisyphilitic drug, 28
Asclepiades, 52

Bacon, Francis, 54
Barbiturates: central nervous system reaction to, 59
Bell, Charles, 60
Boyle, Robert, 84–85
British Pharmaceutical Codex: comparison with *Pharmacopoeia* as standard, 29
British Pharmacopoeia: development as standard, 16–29, 43–46
—nineteenth century: as statutory under Adulteration Acts, 24–25
—1914 edition: effect on drug quality, 27–30; failure to control tablets, 40; legal status, 27–29
British Veterinary Codex, 29
Brockendon, William: patented machine to compress tablets, 40

Capsules, gelatin: industrial development of, 76
Chemistry, Bureau of: and drug examination, 151–54; Notices of Judgment against adulterated food and drugs, 148

Chloramphenicol: FDA advisory committee on, 189; mentioned, 159
Christison, Sir Robert, 10
Citizens' Advisory Committee: supportive criticism to FDA, 164–65
Civil War: impact upon American pharmaceutical industry, 91, 105–11
Code of Federal Regulations, 165–69
Codex medicamentarius sive pharmacopoeia Gallica: absence of assays for identity and purity, 12–14; Commissions for, 11; legal basis for, 10–11; Paris, 1758, attempt to standardize drugs, 3; usefulness of, 11
College of Pharmacy, Paris, 1777: founding, 3
Compressed tablets, 40
Consumer protection: FDA role in, commentary on, 180–85
Council on Pharmacy and Chemistry: changes over the years, 123–31; established by AMA, 113–15; policy changes, commentary on, 135–38; *see also* American Medical Association; Seal of Acceptance program

Depression, Great: effect on drug market, 155–56
Detail men, 140–41
Dieterich, Eugen, 72
Diphtheria antitoxin: industrial development of, 75–76
Dosimetric granule, 76–77
Drug Amendments Act of 1962, 125–26
Drug availability: factors influencing control of industry, 79–82
Drug-import law of 1848, 101, 187
Drug sales after 1930, 171
Drug specifications: *Pharmacopoeia of the United States*, 103–4, 108–10; therapeutic equivalency of, 102–5
Drug testing; *see* Evaluation of drugs

Ego depressants: barbiturates as, 59
Egyptian medicine: survey, 51
Elixir Sulfanilamide tragedy, 158, 165
Epitome of the U.S. Pharmacopoeia and National Formulary, 119
Ethics of experimentation: drug trials, 91–93
Evaluation of drugs: animal experimentation, 55–56, 58, 172; Francis Bacon and, 54; Galen and, 54; on blood in vitro, eighteenth century, 56–57; Paracelsus and, 54; self-experimentation, 58; Zimmerman and, 53, 55–56
—clinical trials: by FDA, 172–74;

eighteenth century, controlled, 56–58; methods unsatisfactory to FDA, 190

Faculty of Medicine, Paris: drug inspection by, 3; mentioned, 4, 11
Fluidextracts: early attempts at drug control, 73; industry taking over pharmacy production of, 72–73
Food and Drug Administration: administrative agency of, quality of, 185; advisory committee of, 189; and Kefauver committees, 193–94; as authorized inspectors of pharmaceutical laboratories, 128; as evaluator of drugs, 126; as reporter of adverse reactions to drugs, 125; assuring communication between drug manufacturer and physician, 168–69; Citizens' Advisory Committee, 164–65; control of prescription vs. over-the-counter drugs, 160–63; criticism of, since 1938, 172–73; effectiveness, 186–88; mentioned, 139; new drug regulations since 1938, 165–68; 1938 to present, progress of, 169–70; proposals for improvement, 189–95; relations with Congress, fiscal appropriations, 163–65; research department, proposal for, 193; role in drug consumer protection, 180–85; supportive role of AMA to, 130–31
Food and Drugs Acts: of 1908, 127; of 1928, British, 34; thalidomide case in violation of, 139
—of 1906: allied federal government with AMA, 115; "drug" defined under, 148; drug supplier's responsibility for drug quality, 107; effects of, 147–56; mentioned, 118, 181; *see also* Sherley Amendment of 1912
Food, Drug and Cosmetic Acts: of 1951, 160–61
—of 1938: discussed, 158–69; mentioned, 130, 171, 181, 182, 186, 188; *see also* Kefauver-Harris Amendments of 1962

Galen: influence on drug therapy, 51, 52, 54
Galenicals: industry taking over pharmacy production of, 72–73
Germinal, Law of, 1803: regulating practice of pharmacy, 5; mentioned, 10
Graduate programs in pharmacy: raised technical specifications for drug quality, 106
Greek medicine: survey, 51–52, 54

Hahnemann, Samuel, 85–86
Hallberg, Carl S. N., 115
Halogens: industry taking over pharmacy
   production of, 73–74
Hassall, Arthur Hill: and microscopy in
   detection of drug adulteration, 16–17,
   21–22; mentioned, 19, 26
Homatropine, 74–75
Humphrey-Durham Amendment, 160–61
Hydrocyanic acid: early problems in
   therapeutic use, 38–39
Hypnotics: barbiturates as, 59

Import Drugs Act of 1848: 101; mentioned, 187
Insulin, 144

*Journal of the American Medical Associa-
tion:* as instructor of proper drug
   therapy, 118–19; criticized for accepting questionable advertisements, 123–
   24; drug advertisements, commentary
   on, 135–36; effects of personnel
   changes, 124–25

Kefauver-Harris Amendments of 1962:
   committee hearings with FDA, 193–
   94; effect on drug costs, 175; effect on
   drug development and control, 173–
   75; effect on new drug approval by
   FDA, 175–76; mentioned, 158

Magendie, Francois, 53, 57, 60
Marshall-Strong Concept, 64
Medicare, 129
Medicines Bill of 1968, British: licensing
   of drugs, 36–37; set up Committee
   on Safety of Drugs, 35–36
Methadone, 136
Mineral drugs: seventeenth, eighteenth,
   and nineteenth centuries, investigators
   of, 9–10
Monthly Index of Medical Specialities, 143
Morphine: for experimental pain, 61–62;
   for pathological pain, 63–64; for tour-
   niquet-induced pain, 67–69

Napoleon: 1810 edict regarding secret
   remedies, 6
National Center for Drug Analysis, 188
National Formulary: comparison with
   Pharmacopoeia of the United States, 109–
   10; mentioned, 111, 125; use as stand-
   ard, 44–46, 115–20 *passim,* 150, 155
National Health Service Act of 1946,
   Britain: drug-testing scheme, 30–31
New and Nonofficial Remedies, 136–37, 141

New drugs: application required by Food,
   Drug and Cosmetic Act of 1938, 159,
   164, 166–67, 183–85; elimination of
   backlog after 1938, 187; FDA methods
   of handling, 172, 175–76; promoting
   use of, 141–42; proposal of "court of
   scientists" for, 189, 190
New York College of Pharmacy: founding, 99

Opium: in theriac, 12
Owen Bill, 120

Pain, quantitative measure of: animal
   experimentation, usefulness of, 62;
   complicated by subjective responses,
   60–70; difference between clinical and
   experimental, 62; difference between
   relief from experimental and large
   doses of narcotic, 61–62; pathological,
   63–64; psychological reaction component of, 64–67; tourniquet-induced,
   67–68
Paracelsus, 52, 54
Patent policies, governmental, 79–80
Penicillin, 159, 171
Pharmaceutical profession: definition, 97
Pharmaceutical Society of Great Britain:
   attention to drug adulteration and control, 20; food and drug analysis, 18;
   mentioned, 25; published *British Pharmaceutical Codex,* 29; published *British
   Veterinary Codex,* 29
Pharmacists: definition of, 97
Pharmacopoeia of the United States: future
   role, 44–46; pharmacists need for, 44–
   45; standard for all drugs, 38–40, 43–
   46, 115, 150, 152, 153, 155; therapeutic
   efficacy of drugs, 43–46
   —contributions to drug quality control:
   1820 edition, 103; 1831 edition, 103–
   4; 1842 edition, 104; 1863 edition,
   105; after 1865, 108–10; mentioned,
   39, 40, 115–21, 141, 144
Pharmacy and Medicines Act of 1941,
   British, 35
Pharmacy departments within state universities, 106
Philadelphia College of Pharmacy, 98–99
Physician-apothecary relationship: influence on drug control, 46
Physiologism: influence on drug therapeutics, 53
Pills: industrial development of, 76
Pilules de Belloste: approval by French
   Academy of Medicine, 7; mentioned,
   5, 6

Placebos: dependence upon stress of effectiveness of, 65–69; effect of mental state on drug, 65–66; effect of situation on drug, 66–67; subjective response to, 61

Plant drugs: seventeenth, eighteenth, and nineteenth centuries, investigators of, 9–10

Police, Paris: surveillance over proprietary medications, 4

Postgate, John: 22–23; mentioned, 19, 21, 26

Poudre de Sency, 7

Prescribers' Journal, 143

Prescription writing: problems in drug control, 42

Proprietary remedies, Paris, 4–6

Psychopharmacology: experimental, 60–70; origins of, 60

Pure Food and Drugs Acts; *see* Food and Drugs acts

Quality control of drugs: Committee on Therapeutic Substances, 31–33; development by pharmaceutical industry, 77–79; needed for better techniques, 177–78

rob Boyveau-Laffecteur, 1764: 4, 6

Royal Society of Medicine, France, 4, 5

Salicylic acid: industrial production of, 74

Salvarsan: discovery of, 28

Scientific progress: commentary on, 88–90

Seal of Acceptance program: commentary, 135–38; dropped by Council on Pharmacy and Chemistry, 123–30; *see also* American Medical Association; Council on Pharmacy and Chemistry

Sedatives: barbiturates as, 59

Sherley Amendment of 1912: enforcement of, 149–50; mentioned, 154; purpose of, 120, 149

Sinclair, Upton, 115

Society of Public Analysts, 25

Sollmann, Torald, 112, 118

Spicers, Paris: comparison with apothecaries, 3

Tablets, compressed, 40, 76

Thalidomide, 139

Therapeutic Substances Act of 1925, British: 33; mentioned, 28

Therapeutic Substances, Committee on Control of, 1920, British: definition of "therapeutic substances," 31–32

Theriac, 12, 46–47

Venereal disease: proprietary remedies for, 4–5

Wakley, Thomas: as crusading editor of *Lancet*, 19, 21–23; mentioned, 26

Wiley, Harvey Washington: as crusader against food adulteration, 147–48; mentioned, 152

World War II, 91, 127

Zimmermann, J. G., 52–56 *passim*

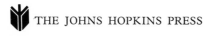 THE JOHNS HOPKINS PRESS

Designed by Edward D. King

Composed in Plantin text and display

*Printed on 60-lb. Perkins and Squier R
by Universal Lithographers, Inc.*

*Bound in Interlaken ARCO Vellum
by L. H. Jenkins Co., Inc.*